PRAISE FOR DOLORES KRIEGER'S THERAPEUTIC TOUCH

"The association between touch and healing is ancient and worldwide. Skilled hands are among the physician's most important diagnostic and therapeutic tools. The importance of touch in medicine has been amply demonstrated . . . in our own time, by nurse/healer Dolores Krieger."

— *The Journal of the American Medical Association*

"A dynamo of a nurse and teacher, [Dolores Krieger] has transformed the practice of laying on of hands into a healing therapy. She has spent years stripping away the aura of mystique, superstition, and suspicion that has confined healing to a select group and opened it up to all."

—*East West/Natural Health*

"Laying on of hands gains new respect!" —*The New York Times*

"Therapeutic Touch has the support of its enthusiasts because their experience indicates that it works. It's a learned procedure whose practitioners report good results." —*Omni*

"There is a quiet revolution taking place in American medicine. The goal: to unite the high-tech wizardry of Western medical approaches with the low-tech, individualized attention of Eastern health care. This union . . . would create a system as strong on prevention as it is on intervention. Under Dr. Krieger's guidance, the technique of Therapeutic Touch has quietly crept into hospital wards throughout the world."

—*Self Magazine*

ACCEPTING
YOUR POWER TO HEAL

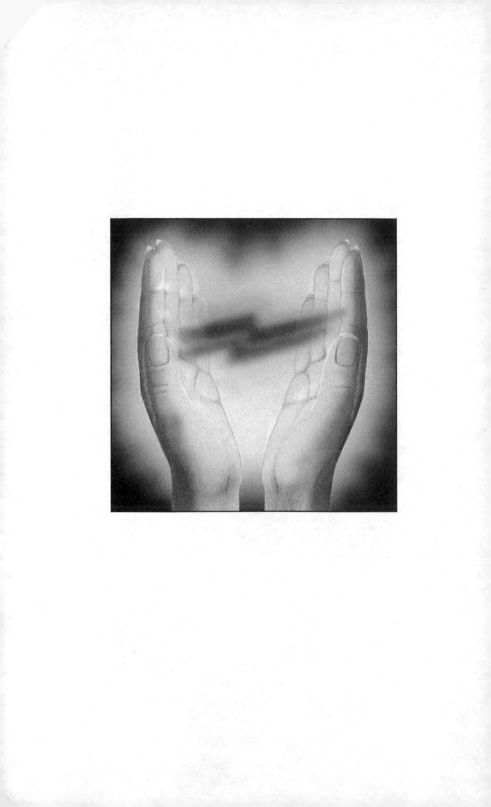

Accepting Your Power to Heal

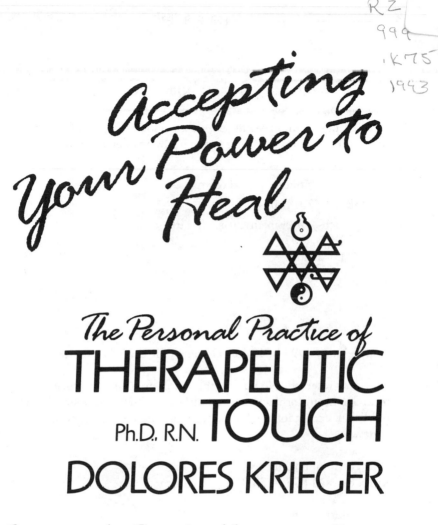

The Personal Practice of
THERAPEUTIC TOUCH

Ph.D. R.N.

DOLORES KRIEGER

Foreword by Stanley Krippner, Ph.D.

BEAR & COMPANY
PUBLISHING
SANTA FE, NEW MEXICO

LIBRARY OF CONGRESS CATALOGING-IN-PUBLICATION DATA
Krieger, Dolores.
    Accepting your power to heal : the personal practice of therapeutic
touch / by Dolores Krieger : foreword by Stanley Krippner.
        p.   cm.
    Includes bibliographical references.
    ISBN 1-879181-04-5
    1.Touch—Therapeutic use. I. Title.
RZ999.K75 1993
615.8′51—dc20   92-42936
                                                           CIP

Bear & Company, Inc.
Santa Fe, NM 87504-2860

Cover illustration: James Finnell © 1993
Cover & interior design: Angela Werneke
Text illustration: Patricia Stewart © 1993
Photos: figure 1 by Diane J. Mancino,
figure 2 by Suzanne Brintzenhofe, figure 11 by Carl Zapp
Title page graphic: "Timeless Mandala" by Dolores Krieger
Editing: Gail Vivino
Typography: Buffalo Publications
Printed in the United States of America by R.R. Donnelley

9 8

To the generations of "Krieger's Krazies"—
may your tribes increase!

Reflections on Therapeutic Touch

I have reached for you in so many ways
one of which was to run
at speeds so fast
I seemed to stand still
while you danced around me.

Now, caressing invisible forces
passing through your energy field,
I've discovered the tempo
and dance to your beauty
which is mine.

—Linda Mowad,
M.A., R.N., Krieger's Krazy

CONTENTS

The Basis of Therapeutic Touch

A Definition of Therapeutic Touch. What Therapeutic Touch Can
Do. Therapeutic Touch for Everyone. Functional Aspects of
Therapeutic Touch. Centering: Getting to Know Yourself.
*Experiential Exercise 1: How to Center. Experiential Exercise 2:
The Luminous Child and the Lake of Quietude.* Assessing the Human
Energy Field. *Experiential Exercise 3: Feeling the Human Energy
Field.* The Assessment Technique. *Experiential Exercise 4: Basic
Techniques for Assessment of the Human Energy Field.* Recognizing
Cues in the Healee's Energy Field. *Experiential Exercise 5: The
Emperor's Clothes.* Assessing the Healee's Energy Field for Emotional
Content. *Experiential Exercise 6: Sensing the Emotions.* In-Depth
Assessment of the Human Energy Field.

The Nature of Human Support Systems. *Experiential Exercise 7:
Directing Human Energy.* Putting the Treatment Together. Major
Techniques of Therapeutic Touch. The Conscious Direction of
Human Energies. *Experiential Exercise 8: Directing Energy Through
the Healee.* Modulating Human Energies. *Experiential Exercise 9:
Appreciating the Energetic Characteristics of Color.* Changing
Patterns in the Human Energy Field. Conventions and Cautions.

Working with a Partner. Systems Most Sensitive to Therapeutic Touch. The Most Reliable Effects of Therapeutic Touch. Personal Experiences with Therapeutic Touch Practice. Putting It Together. *Experiential Exercise 10: Post-Assessment Data Sheet and Healee Evaluation Form.*

A Systems Model for the Therapeutic Touch Assessment. Allies in the Healing Process. The Concept of Human Energy. The Experience of Therapeutic Touch. *Experiential Exercise 11: The Human Barrier Game.* The Search for Ordering Principles. Table I: Close Relationships. Table II: Visualized Protective Barriers.

How Therapeutic Touch Has Been Used. Pregnancy. Labor and Delivery. Postnatal Treatment. Pain. Premenstrual Syndrome (PMS). Helping Persons Who Are HIV+. Abdominal Operations and Caesarian Sections. How You Know. *Experiential Exercise 12: Using the Hand Chakras to Rebalance the Healee's Energy Field.* Other Examples of Therapeutic Touch in Practice. A Few Suggestions. Cautions and Precautions. Legal Implications.

The Context of Therapeutic Touch Practice. The Centering Phase. The Assessment Phase. The Rebalancing Phase. Chakras. Conjoint Practices. *Experiential Exercise 13: The Nature of Therapeutic Touch.* The Miracle of Therapeutic Touch.

ILLUSTRATIONS

ACKNOWLEDGMENTS

Therapeutic Touch started out as the focus of my first major postdoctoral research, and the development of my first tentative queries into Therapeutic Touch became the challenge for my life's work. In the past twenty-five years, many people have been helpful to me personally and to the expression of Therapeutic Touch, people whom I am happy to acknowledge at this time.

Foremost, I would like to acknowledge the deeply thoughtful collaboration and guidance of my colleague Dora Kunz. As this book goes to press, we celebrate the twentieth anniversary of our initial development of Therapeutic Touch. Without her impress, the continuing development and refinement of this system would have been less significant to the understanding of the healing process and less sensitive to the subtle implications for both healer and healee during the healing process. And certainly, the conceiving of Therapeutic Touch would have been much less fun!

Stanley Krippner, Ph.D., who is recognized as a world authority for his distinguished studies on the dynamics of the farther reaches of mind, has honored me in writing the foreword to *Accepting Your Power to Heal,* and I offer him my deep appreciation.

Throughout this time, Nabeela George was an ever-ready, perceptive sounding board for clarity of ideas. She offered assurance that they translated into commonsensical, minimally syllabic word structures, and her light grounding touch is much appreciated.

The acceptance of Therapeutic Touch has benefited immeasurably from the consistent support of college and university faculties in the United States and abroad, of professional organizations in the health field, and of progressive groups with alternative and complementary approaches to healing and helping such as is the Nurse Healers-Professional Associates, Inc.

Not least is my appreciation for the generations of my students, who call themselves "Krieger's Krazies." They have always been willing to challenge me to think more clearly and deeply and to say things more simply. So, thanks—like, y'know what I mean?

This book itself would have been but an amalgam of words and ideas without the artful shaping and considered sculpting of Barbara Clow, Barbara Doern Drew, Gail Vivino, and the rest of the professional staff at Bear & Company.

FOREWORD

Dolores Krieger is one of the contemporary pioneers in integrating the spiritual dimension of healing with mainstream professional nursing practices. Over the past decades, she has developed "Therapeutic Touch" (or TT), a creative interpretation of several ancient healing practices that deal with such concepts as the "laying-on" of hands, "energy transfer," and the "inner healer." As professor of nursing at New York University, Dr. Krieger has been able to conduct research, teach students, and develop the technique and philosophy of TT. Ultimately, Therapeutic Touch has been taught in more than eighty colleges and universities in the United States and in more than seventy foreign countries, especially in schools of nursing.

In the 1980s, I took a copy of Dr. Krieger's first book on Therapeutic Touch, *The Therapeutic Touch: How to Use Your Hands to Help or to Heal,* to the former Soviet Union. It immediately passed into the underground press and was translated, typed, copied, and passed from hand to hand. It even made its way into Poland and some of the Eastern European countries.

Dr. Krieger deserves credit for initiating research with Therapeutic Touch and for encouraging other researchers to attempt replication of her findings. Although the practice is still a matter of controversy, there is enough supportive data so that Therapeutic Touch must be taken seriously by informed practitioners. Whether TT involves 'energy transfer' is an open question, as is the role played by expectation and rapport. Nevertheless, Dr. Krieger's concepts of "energy congestion" and "energy imbalance" can certainly be considered useful metaphors that refer to the mechanisms involved, processes that may eventually be understood by new developments in the field of psychoneuroimmunology, which explores mind-body relationships.

A client's behavior is of primary importance to Dr. Krieger, who tells her students to listen to nuances in the voice, to observe breathing patterns, and to be aware of the use of unusual language in the description of symptoms. She also attempts to learn about a client's spiritual problems, concerns, and beliefs, and how they may impact treatment. The prime goal of Therapeutic Touch is the alleviation of discomfort and the acceleration of the client's self-healing capacities; spiritual orientation may be a key element in the attainment of these ends.

Members of the entire spectrum of the health professions have incorporated Therapeutic Touch into their practices; practitioners have a wide variety of orientations, including allopathic, osteopathic, chiropractic, naturopathic, and homeopathic. Dr. Krieger's new book, *Accepting Your Power to Heal: The Personal Practice of Therapeutic Touch*, expands her audience from these healing professionals to include all people who have an interest in tapping their own powers of healing and using them.

In this book, Dr. Krieger presents the basic TT concepts, following them with experiential exercises that bring these abstractions to life. These imaginative activities are clearly described, and they are discussed in a manner that is both wise and practical. For example, Dr. Krieger admonishes, "If you don't know, don't do." She also cites the modalities with which TT can be paired, for example, acupressure, massage, mental imagery, physical therapy, and yoga.

Dr. Krieger divides the major effects of TT into four categories: relaxation, pain reduction, accelerated healing, and the alleviation of psychosomatic symptoms. Not all healees will experience each of these phenomena, but any of them would be appreciated by most individuals suffering from major and minor illnesses. These phenomena are all the more welcome when one considers that TT is remarkably nonintrusive and that it is a basic human capacity that can be learned and practiced by thoughtful, disciplined laypeople as well as by health-care workers. I believe that TT can also be beneficial to the healers themselves, allowing them to become more aware of their own mind and body processes while they direct their compassion toward helping those in pain or discomfort.

Dr. Krieger has lost none of her pioneering orientation over the years. Nor has she lost her ability to stimulate controversy! *Accepting Your Power to Heal* boldly leaps beyond the current parameters of TT, discussing implications for the frontiers of medicine and for the health care of the future. The ideas and processes put forward in this book most probably will still be debated, discussed, and (most important) practiced in the decades to come.

Stanley Krippner, Ph.D.
San Francisco, California
October 1992

Stanley Krippner is a distinguished professor of psychology at the California School of Integral Studies and professor of psychology at Saybrook Institute. He is the coauthor of Spiritual Dimensions of Healing, Personal Mythology, Dreamworking, *and* Healing States.

PREFACE

Accepting Your Power to Heal can be used as a guide for individual practice, for coordinated practice of Therapeutic Touch between two persons, or for practice within a group. In all instances, it is for helping or healing those who are ill.

The text has been designed for use in formal curriculums, informal workshops, or independent study. The format of the exercises ensures progressive knowledge about the Therapeutic Touch process and graded experiences in its practice.

The substantive discussions are designed to explore assumptions and implications of the process per se and to prepare the reader for the nature of the therapeutic interactional experiences. Some experiences are transpersonal; all offer to the reader the possibility of actualizing individual potential for personal growth during a quest for understanding one of the most humane of all human endeavors.

A number of graphic illustrations demonstrate the techniques of Therapeutic Touch. Several exercises explore through guided imagery the "feel" or mood that accompanies the knowledgeable and compassionate use of the human energy field to help or heal others who are in need. Appendix II offers a standardized system for measuring over time one's ability to practice Therapeutic Touch.

*Accepting
Your Power to
Heal*

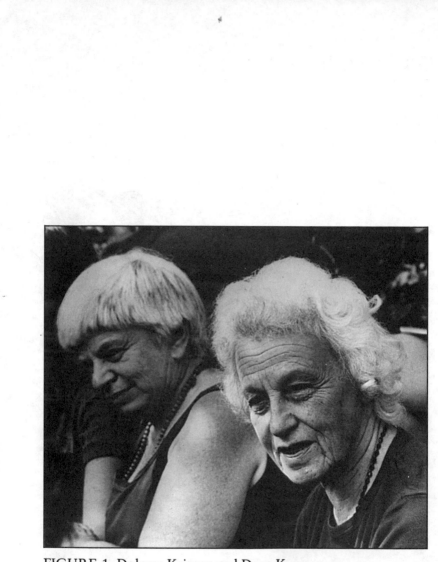

FIGURE 1. Dolores Krieger and Dora Kunz

Chapter 1

AN INTRODUCTION
TO THERAPEUTIC TOUCH

I reached forward and, with a click, put an end to the crackle of static on the car radio. My attention turned to the wind-driven sheets of rain that were picked out of the dark night by the bright headlights. I was on the first leg of a cross-country automobile trip that had started much later in the day than I had initially intended. However, I was not tired, and as I drove, the rhythmic beat of the windshield wipers blended with the soft glow of the dashboard lights, creating a comfortable atmosphere.

The traffic was very light and undemanding of my full involvement, so as my car turned into a wide curve on the road, I had ample opportunity to consider a sign pointing to the emergency room of a local hospital. Most of the lights in the hospital's rooms were out at this late hour, but, as my eyes scanned the scene unfolding before the glare of the car's headlights, I noticed the unmistakable large skylight of a surgical operating room in the uppermost story of the building.

Oh yes, I said to myself, it's time for the night shift; Marianne will be working up there. Marianne was one of my former students. Looking up at the blue-bright fluorescence shining clearly through the skylight and challenging the darkness of that stormy night, my mind conjured up several scenarios of Marianne's activities.

Some years ago, in a class at a major university, I had taught Marianne a contemporary interpretation of ancient healing practices that I had named Therapeutic Touch. Therapeutic Touch is a healing practice based on the conscious use of the hands to direct

3

or modulate, for therapeutic purposes, selected nonphysical human energies that activate the physical body. My colleague Dora Kunz and I had initiated the development of Therapeutic Touch in 1972 specifically for persons in the health professions, and Marianne was one of several thousands of nurses who had learned it from us. Over the years, Marianne and I had kept up an active correspondence, and I knew that she had continued to practice Therapeutic Touch as an extension of her professional skills.

Considering the many ways in which she might be using Therapeutic Touch in the operating theater, I remember that Marianne had teamed up with Ellen, another student who now was a county public-health nurse. Together they assured that there would be follow-ups of Therapeutic Touch treatments for patients who were discharged from the hospital. Ellen taught the patients' relatives the basic techniques of Therapeutic Touch so that treatments would be uninterrupted, if they were still needed. Marianne and Ellen were but one of several health-care teams throughout the country whose members incorporated Therapeutic Touch into their professional practices.

Within the line of my peripheral vision, I could see a road map lying on the seat by my side, my proposed journey marked in red. I had planned to drive through the night, and as I reviewed my intended progress westward, I recalled other former students who might be at work in health facilities in the various states I would be passing through on the way to my first stop. They might be doing Therapeutic Touch even as I drove through their towns.

As I left Massachusetts, I would pass by the hospital where Jean taught husbands to do Therapeutic Touch on their pregnant wives. Further south, in Connecticut, there was Faith, who, like Marianne, also used Therapeutic Touch in an operating room. In New York, there were many professional persons engaged in Therapeutic Touch practice. I knew that Carol would be working with terminally ill patients, using Therapeutic Touch techniques to ameliorate pain and provide a respite from the anxiety and agitation of sleepless nights. This respite would occur through the relaxation response that accompanies treatment by Therapeutic Touch.

As my car skirted New York City, Joanne, at work in the inner city, would be using Therapeutic Touch to relieve her tiny charges in the intensive-care nursery of a large medical center. When I crossed the Hudson River into New Jersey, Sue would be finishing up her all-night crisis clinic at a psychiatric center not far from the turnpike on which I would be traveling. She had incorporated Therapeutic Touch into her psychotherapy work and had taught the practice to many other therapists in surrounding towns. Perhaps I would call her from a nearby phone and we could have coffee together. Or, I might slip into Philadelphia to escape the early traffic and have coffee with Danny before he donned his clown's garb and went to the pediatric hospital. There, he would creatively intermix Therapeutic Touch with his clowning antics to add the precious ingredient of laughter to the children's treatments.

The Basis of Therapeutic Touch

In the two decades since Dora Kunz and I first began the development of Therapeutic Touch, I myself have taught this useful technique to more than thirty-six thousand professional persons in the health-care field, and I am sure that Ms. Kunz has taught again as many. At the time of this writing (1990), Therapeutic Touch has also been taught in more than eighty colleges and universities in the United States, as well as in innumerable hospital and health facility in-service and continuing education programs. In addition, Therapeutic Touch has been taught in sixty-eight countries. (See appendix 1.)

The transcultural and transpersonal nature of Therapeutic Touch has been attested to by its use in many of the stress-filled locations of today's world. To name but a few: Therapeutic Touch has been used by both Egyptians and Israelis during the fighting in the Gaza Strip; in South Africa, it has been used by both blacks and whites—among themselves and on each other; it has flourished in the Underground in both the former Soviet Union and in Poland; and, through a group of doctors, nurses, and other former students who volunteered to work in a Cambodian refugee camp called Ghouy Dang, in Thailand, it has been recognized by Cambodian patients as being closely akin to their own native practices.

Why so much interest in Therapeutic Touch? Part of the answer, I believe, lies in our continuing ignorance about the causes of many human illnesses in spite of our high-tech expertise. The simple healing practice of Therapeutic Touch, involving only the explicit, conscious direction and modulation of natural human energies, has demonstrated its usefulness with a wide variety of illnesses. Also, science is the reality that Western civilization accepts. It is based on rational theory derived from formal research that requires rigorous replication before research findings are accepted. The development of Therapeutic Touch has respected these criteria. Much of the basis of its practice has been drawn from a substantive body of basic and clinical research that has continued throughout the past twenty years.

Perhaps more significant to the widespread interest in Therapeutic Touch is the fact that cross-cultural communication systems (that science itself has produced) have led to the realization that there is not only one reality, or even specified "alternate" realities, that satisfy all the conditions for reality among the many cultures of our global village, Earth. It is now recognized that the concept of multiple realities is valid; a particular view of reality is dependent only upon the particular facet of human consciousness that is permitted to operate at the time.

Within this universe of multiple realities, illness can have many connotations. Several views of reality do not perceive illness as "bad"; rather, they see illness as an individual's reaction to circumstances. Within this context, an illness can be helped or healed by the individual him- or herself through appropriate self-stimulation of the enzymes in the brain. Subjective experiences that can spark such self-healing have served to broaden the idea of placebo response. Since it cannot be ruled out that the highly personalized interaction that goes on between the Therapeutic Touch practitioner and the client does not create a placebo response to the expectation of healing, Therapeutic Touch has benefited by being perceived in this more liberal perspective.

In fact, a basic recognition upon which Therapeutic Touch was developed initially was exactly that, in the final analysis, it is the healee (client) who heals her- or himself. The healer or therapist, in this view, acts as a human energy support system until the healee's own immunological system is robust enough to take over.

Over the years, experience gained from the continued use of Therapeutic Touch has served to demonstrate that it can be used safely and effectively not only by health-field professionals but by laypeople who are committed to helping or healing persons in need. However, commitment, like love, in itself is not enough. Important additional qualities that are needed include: compassion; a sensitive, balanced receptivity to the unstated and often unrecognized nonphysical needs of the healee; a readiness to discipline oneself to finely attune the inner "antennae" by which the messages coming from the farther reaches of consciousness can become available; and, not least, the willingness to recognize honestly and objectively one's own human limitations.

Given these qualities, after a short period of consistent use of Therapeutic Touch (our records indicate that two to three weeks is the average) the practitioner will be able to elicit in the healee the following therapeutic changes:

- A well-developed general relaxation response within the first five minutes of therapy.
- Very frequently a significant reduction in, or cessation of, painful symptoms during the therapeutic session, which usually lasts twenty to twenty-five minutes.
- An acceleration of the healing process in appropriate cases.

As shall be clarified in the following pages, these therapeutic changes are highly reliable and occur with remarkable consistency in the basic, formal, and clinical research done by myself and my students and colleagues over the past two decades.

In conclusion, the final answer to the question of why there is so much interest in Therapeutic Touch is that Therapeutic Touch works. It can be helpful to persons with a wide range of illnesses, as attested to by a growing body of substantive research findings. This book has been written so that you, the reader, will realize a highly reliable and useful aspect of yourself that can be intelligently used to help or heal those in need. Healing is a natural potential that can be actualized under the appropriate circumstances. You can do it; everyone who is willing to undertake the discipline to learn Therapeutic Touch can do it. You need only try in order to determine the truth of this statement for yourself. So, I invite you: TRY.

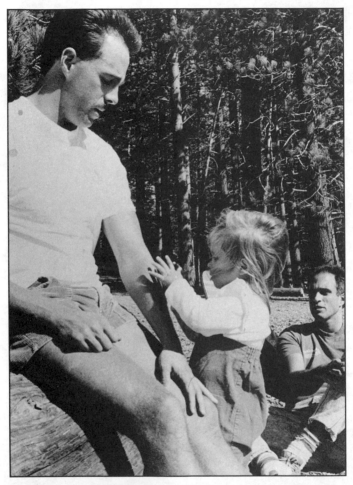
FIGURE 2. Child Administering Therapeutic Touch to Her Uncle

chapter 2

BASIC TECHNIQUES OF THERAPEUTIC TOUCH

A Definition of Therapeutic Touch

Therapeutic Touch is a contemporary interpretation of several ancient healing practices. These practices consist of learned skills for consciously directing or sensitively modulating human energies. The term *Therapeutic Touch* may in fact be a misnomer because, in practice, the healer need not make physical contact with the patient (healee). Much of the work done by the person playing the role of healer has as its primary focus the modulation of the healee's energy field rather than the touch or manipulation of his or her skin.

Suggestion can act as an ever-present and powerful placebo in human healing interactions. However, the responses to Therapeutic Touch are not solely or overtly due to suggestion or persuasion. Some of the most startling therapeutic responses have occurred in persons not thought capable of responding to verbal command, such as premature babies, postoperative patients who have been deeply anesthetized, and persons who are in coma and unaware of their surroundings.

Neither is Therapeutic Touch a miracle cure; it is simply an opportunity to actualize the natural human potential to help or heal yourself or others. Over the past twenty years, as Dora Kunz and I developed Therapeutic Touch, there were several basic scientific assumptions that guided our rationale. Following are four of these scientific premises.

- *All the life sciences agree that, physically, a human being is an open energy system.* This assumption implies that the transfer of energy between people is a natural, continuous event. Therefore, when a healer transfers energy to a healee during Therapeutic Touch, it is by a nonstressful, "effortless effort" that is guided by conscious, mindful action. The important ingredient added by the healer is *intentionality* within a context of compassionate concern for the healee.

- *Anatomically, a human being is bilaterally symmetrical.* This symmetry is apparent in both the circulatory and the neural nets. However, the characteristic bilateral balance of form is most clearly seen in the human skeleton, with its mirrorlike reflection of bone construction on either side of the longitudinal axis of the spinal column. This symmetry is the rational basis for inferring that there is also a pattern in the underlying human energy field. This assumption is the background for the Therapeutic Touch practitioner's assessment of the healee's energy state.

- *Illness is an imbalance in an individual's energy field.* In Therapeutic Touch, the healer directs and modulates this energy field, using the sense of touch as a telereceptor, much like the other four major senses of the body. All of these senses can act over distance without connecting apparatus: sight via photons; taste and smell by means of chemical molecules; hearing through acoustical pressures; and touch, for the Therapeutic Touch practitioner, via fine energetic cues such as changes in pattern. These cues occur in the human energy field that extends a few inches from the body surface of the person being treated. They can also be sensed through direct contact with the person's skin.

- *Human beings have natural abilities to transform and*

transcend their conditions of living. In a sense, these functions are the necessary prerequisites for healing to occur.

The practice of Therapeutic Touch is based upon these assumptions. You as the healer act as a human support system, your own healthy energy field providing the scaffolding to guide the repatterning of the healee's weakened and disrupted energy flow. Such support is oriented toward stimulating the healee's own immunological system, for, in the final analysis, it is the healee who heals her- or himself.

In Therapeutic Touch, the healing act per se is a conscious act, in contradistinction to a passive, trancelike, or hypnagogic state. This healing act is based upon a body of knowledge derived from logical deduction, formal and clinical research findings, the compendium of world literature concerning the therapeutic use of human energies, and deep experiential knowledge that grows into a personal knowing.

What Therapeutic Touch Can Do

There are several consistent and highly reliable results of the Therapeutic Touch interaction:

- **Relaxation.** The first response of the healee is a very rapid relaxation response, in many instances occurring in as little as two to four minutes.
- **Pain reduction.** Clinically, there is a significant amelioration or eradication of pain. In many cases, this occurs when analgesics are no longer effective for ill persons. Many terminally ill patients, once freed from the stress of persistent pain, are able to go on to a peaceful transition into death.
- **Accelerated healing process.** Primarily because the relaxation response and the relief from pain have salutary effects on the healee's immunological system, Therapeutic Touch accelerates the healing process. One of the clearest ex-

amples of this is the healing of bone fractures. With Therapeutic Touch, good callus formation (the precursor to bone development) can be seen in x-rays in approximately two and a half weeks, rather than the six weeks it usually takes.

• **Alleviation of psychosomatic illness.** Of the physiological systems that are sensitive to Therapeutic Touch, my choice for the most sensitive is the autonomic nervous system. Therapeutic Touch deals best with many of this system's dysfunctions, which are at the heart of what are known as psychosomatic illnesses. Society once looked askance at these illnesses, but today it is recognized that up to 70 percent of the illnesses in the world are psychosomatic in origin. This is because stress-related illnesses are pandemic, even in Third-World countries. It is the sensitivity of the autonomic nervous system to Therapeutic Touch that creates the consistent and rapid relaxation response.

Therapeutic Touch for Everyone

In many hospitals, teams of nurses as well as interdisciplinary teams use Therapeutic Touch in their daily clinical practices. From one such group in Canada, a nurse recently wrote:

> I was traveling the road near Brandon (Manitoba) the other day when I saw the flashing lights of a police car near the site of an accident. I pulled over and walked to the cars, thinking to help by doing Therapeutic Touch to any of the accident victims who might need it. However, when I got to the area I saw that David, a pediatrician on our team at the hospital, had gotten there before me and already was doing Therapeutic Touch to one of the drivers.

In this instance, the nurse and physician worked together on the side of the road, in the intermittent glare of the red, flashing lights of the police vehicle. They did Therapeutic Touch as first aid to the wounded until an ambulance arrived and emergency equipment was put in place. They then turned their attention to other passengers who were still shocked by their involvement in the traumatic accident. Through the relaxation response rapidly elicited by Therapeutic Touch, they succeeded in helping the passengers regain control of themselves.

Therapeutic Touch has also reached deeply into the community. In several parts of the United States, senior citizens, particularly those known as the Grey Panthers, have developed local programs that I call "peer therapeutics." They regularly visit nursing homes and other sites for people of comparable age and treat them with Therapeutic Touch.

Therapeutic Touch is used freely within families as a means for family members to care for one another. In one family, a newly married couple was in an accident in which the young wife suffered extensive damage to her knees. The agonized husband and the wife's mother stood at the foot of the bed after the wife's operation. She had been heavily sedated, but even as she slept they watched her face twist in grimaces that reflected her continued pain. Rather than stand by helplessly, they moved around to the side of her bed and did Therapeutic Touch to her. Within a short time, they were delighted to see a grin slowly spread over her face, and when they left for the night she was deeply and quietly asleep. For another example of Therapeutic Touch use in families, see figure 2.

It would seem, without a doubt, that Therapeutic Touch is indeed for everyone. Therefore, I invite you to join me in the next several chapters as I discuss how you, too, can learn to help or heal with Therapeutic Touch. The basic techniques are not only simple, they are natural. The more advanced techniques, I assure you, will lead you into a most intriguing study of yourself, for Therapeutic Touch is an interior experience, a seeking within. As you make these techniques your own, there will be an upwelling of the further reaches of your own consciousness. Through this process, the empowerment to help or heal yourself and others will arise.

Functional Aspects of Therapeutic Touch

In practice, Therapeutic Touch is concerned with the knowledgeable use of the therapeutic functions of the human energy field. This is in contradistinction to traditional medical diagnosis, which is a highly sophisticated classification system that is important within its own context. Within this latter system, Therapeutic Touch is inappropriate. Therapeutic Touch is a primitive, simple (that is, direct), and elegant use of human energies in the service of a humane act. It is from compassion that it draws its power. Therefore, I will leave a more intellectual discussion of the dynamics of the human energy field to a later chapter and begin by considering human energy from a functional standpoint.

In our culture, energy is classically defined as a force that does work. Energy, however, is multifaceted and takes on many guises—for example, the pressured energy of steam that forces a heavy cogwheel to turn, or the light brush of my fingertips on computer keys to quietly store words I am writing "in the electricity," or a nonmaterial energy field that I cannot see or taste or smell. Energy, however, is not only a workhorse for things mechanical. Humans, too, are energetic beings. Human emotions do work, as measured, for instance, in the responsive body sweat tallied by the galvanic skin response. Human thoughts do work as measured by magnetoencephalographic readings.

It is in the brain that the various patterns and levels of energy become meaningful. Hands, which are the major physical instruments of Therapeutic Touch, seem to be the prime stimuli-seeking extensions of the brain. Healing, which is the foremost function of Therapeutic Touch, could be called a humanization of energy in the interest of helping or healing others or oneself. The first thing you do when learning Therapeutic Touch, and frequently the major factor for learning it, is to heal yourself, which is proper and perhaps even necessary.

Centering: Getting to Know Yourself

The point of entry into the Therapeutic Touch process is the act of "centering" your consciousness. Centering is an act of self-searching, a going within to explore the deeper levels of yourself. In this act of journeying inward, you can learn, like a yogi, to trace or follow the energy flows of your own consciousness in a quest to understand your own being and your relationship to the universe.

The importance of centering is the fact that, in Therapeutic Touch, you, as the healer, are the sole determiner of what will happen during the therapeutic process. It is you who initiates the interaction. How the process proceeds depends upon your ability to discriminate among the subtle cues of the healee's energy-field dynamics. Finally, it is your considered judgment that will decide when the Therapeutic Touch process is to be terminated and how this shall occur. The insubstantiality of the energy flows that you are dealing with makes it imperative that you feel quite sure of your judgments, which are largely subjective in nature.

In centering your consciousness, you go beyond the everyday stimulus and response of bodily interactions with the environment, or the world "out there." In centering, you relate to the extraordinary stillness of the personal, private world within you, and you bask in its profoundly quieting psychological and physical effects. In time, you begin to realize that you are your consciousness. You perceive that the way you color and give substance to your experiences is through the relationships you build between yourself and other beings or things or ideas. You may start to appreciate the necessity of clearly acknowledging these relationships without previous bias.

During Therapeutic Touch, this centering process translates into a respect for the individuality of each person's dynamics. You can then bring to a moment everything in your past experience that might help meet a person's needs in a therapeutic manner.

In general, healing might be described as the conscious, full engagement of your energies in the interest of helping another. With Therapeutic Touch, this interest arises from a sense of compassion and a recognition that there is an underlying order in the universe. This learning occurs experientially through the process of centering. In Therapeutic Touch, you not only start the healing process by centering your consciousness, but you then stay on center throughout the entirety of the healing enactment. This sounds very difficult. However, although it demands concentration, it is a very enjoyable experience, because in centering you are learning about the dynamics of your own consciousness.

In this act of quietude, you can ask questions. Then, if you listen very carefully, quite profound answers can be reflected from the deep places of your inner self. It is not easy to still the chattering "monkey brain" and focus your attention on the responses that well up from the deep reaches of your consciousness. However, if your motivation is high enough, a way will be found in a surprisingly short time.

EXPERIENTIAL EXERCISE 1

How to Center

1. Start simply. Sit in a comfortable position and take quiet, full breaths. It does not matter whether or not your eyes are closed. The purpose is to become aware of the fullness of your own being.

2. Be aware of what you feel like when you are quiet. Explore your own being and notice feelings that edge into your consciousness. Quietly follow thoughts that cross your mind without getting too emotionally involved in them.

3. From amongst the energies you perceive, distinguish which ones belong to you and which ones belong to other things or people with whom you may be identifying. Concentrate on your own attributes.

4. As you gain a sense of self, become sensitive to your own more subtle energies. You can begin by quietly becoming aware of your own breathing, noticing how your breath fills your lungs. Then try to sense how your breath permeates the tissues of your body and quickens its functioning with life-sustaining prana, or vital energy. Now shift your attention to take note of other subtle energies. If someone else is in the room, how do you sense his or her presence? If something distracts your attention, can you capture the process of visualization that brings it to your attention? Can you follow the process of how you feel an emotion for someone who is not physically present?

5. As you gain facility with this exercise, try to go one step further. Attempt to identify, by mood or feeling, with the facet of your consciousness that senses energies and creates visualizations or emotions. As you access these deeper levels of your being, you will become aware of an enveloping stillness and a sense of timelessness. In this stillness, you will not find it difficult to attain a state of receptivity in which personal insights may emerge. You may find it useful to have a pen and pad at hand so that you can jot down key thoughts or symbols without disturbing your train of thought.

You will have stepped into another, often unrealized dimension of yourself, and, in actuality, you will not notice the deep quietude or sense of timelessness until you come off center. At that moment, you also will feel a sense of well-being, relaxation, and being in command of yourself. This is a very nice feeling, and you will look forward to repeating the experience.

Comments on Exercise 1

It is important to know your own center so that you can help others reach theirs. As you learn to quiet the inner turmoil of meaningless dialogue with your "monkey brain," you can more clearly heed your psyche's answers to your questions. Moreover, when you thoroughly understand this tranquil state, you will find that you can use it during Therapeutic Touch processing. From this state of consciousness, you can treat clients for a wide range of disorders, including irritability, restlessness, anxiety, hypertension, chemotherapy sickness, and inflammatory disease processes. The treatment will occur in a manner that may not be meaningful to you now but will become more so by the time you have finished this chapter.

Centering experiences range widely, from the grounded feeling of physical centeredness to awareness of the transcendent functions of consciousness. As the process of centering is experienced over time, it brings the various aspects of the human energy field into resonance with one another. It integrates the various facets of the personality. You then feel more of one piece, more focused. You know with a personal surety that when engagement of the self is a conscious act, there can be a redirection (or transformation) of the personality. Out of this realization, your sense of the future becomes more life affirming. The sum of these insights leads to the personal knowledge that this act of quietude provides access to the inner self, the teacher, the guide, who is a reflection of your individual power.

To simulate the sense of stillness and timelessness characteristic of the centering experience and, in addition, create a situation in which you can observe the dynamics of the visualization process, you may wish to use the guided imagery offered in Experiential Exercise 2.

EXPERIENTIAL EXERCISE 2

The Luminous Child and the Lake of Quietude

All techniques to center your consciousness are marked by a characteristic atmosphere of pervading stillness; this sense of quietude is ever-present. To do the following guided imagery, either have somebody slowly read it to you while you close your eyes and follow the imagery, or read the exercise into a tape recorder and then play it back to yourself. In order for this exercise to be effective, there must be adequate pauses throughout it in order to give you ample time to conjure up in your mind the suggested imagery. However, the pauses should not be so prolonged that you lose the thread of imagery continuity.

Do not program the experience. Let every moment of it tell you its own story, and listen to it quietly. Think of it as an experience to enjoy and to learn from, as you would learn from a friend.

Procedure

Sit in a comfortable position, one hand on your lower abdomen. Center your consciousness. Slow down and gentle your breath until you feel your lower abdomen respond and become as still as a lake of utter quietude.

There is not a ripple on the lake. Look for an area of it that is shining. Can you see a pattern of light in that area of the quiet lake?

Look closely at this pattern and notice that there is a childlike figure in the shining light. This figure is neither human nor nonhuman; it is just a childlike figure that depicts a sense of innocent acceptance and simple serenity. Don't expect or program this figure to be anything in particular; just allow it to be on its own terms.

Sensitively expand your own energy field and feel the presence of the figure. Match its breathing pattern. Trust it and identify with it, for it is of your own nature.

Ahead of you, see the glistening lake. Step into the lake and take the hand of the luminous child by touching it with the energy center that overlies the space just above the palm of your hand.

The child's touch is as light as a butterfly. Stay sensitive to this light touch and ask it to show you how to understand it.

Now, feel at one with your deepest wish or commitment to help others and clearly form a question in your mind. Ask the question of the child presence and then let it go as gently as a feathery fluff floating on the breeze.

Listen carefully.

Do not allow the surface of the lake to ruffle; keep the surface calm and undisturbed. Use slow, deep breaths to clear away pockets of tension.

The touch of your luminous child is like cool, flowing water on the placid surface of the lake. An answer comes to you that is as clear and refreshing as the touch of the waters.

After you receive your answer, take a deep breath and very slowly open your eyes.

Know that this experience is only the beginning. There will be other times and other experiences.

Assessing the Human Energy Field

It is from a state of centeredness that you can proceed with the rest of the Therapeutic Touch process. At first, you may find it unusual to be doing more than one thing at a time. However, let me assure you that this is a very natural thing to do, and you do it many times a day. The difference is that now you are doing it consciously.

Once you are centered, the next step is to understand the situation before you by engaging in an assessment or evaluation of the healee's energy field. The prime assumption here is that human beings are open energy systems: we do not stop at our skins. The human energy system flows unimpeded and intermixes with other energies in a process that is always in flux. Moreover, physical exertion is not necessary to assure this natural flow. This suggests that transfer of energy from one individual's system to another's can occur effortlessly. In Therapeutic Touch, this energy flow is effortlessly directed or modulated in specific, appropriate ways by the knowledgeable use of the mind.

Therapeutic Touch is a conscious act; nothing is done on impulse. There is always a good reason or a strong, irresistible, intuitive urge for using particular Therapeutic Touch techniques. The healing act per se is cue specific. The cues (to energy imbalances) are recognized during the assessment phase.

Therefore, in order to act in a knowledgeable manner, you must first have some idea of what is the matter with the healee from a human-energy perspective. To do this, remember the second basic assumption of Therapeutic Touch, noted previously: The physical body exhibits bilateral symmetry, with the left and right sides of the body anatomically reflecting each other.

This premise allows you to search out imbalances in the ill person's energy field. Essentially, if the energy field in health is symmetrical and if, as the third assumption states, illness is characterized by an energy field that is not in balance, then you can find areas of energy deficit or illness by searching out signs of asymmetry in the healee's energy field.

However, what does a human energy field feel like? According to the findings of the East Indians, there are certain nonphysical transformers of energy called *chakras* that are within the human energy field. All human beings have and use these chakras, whether we are aware of them or not, for they are in fact centers of different levels of consciousness, ranging from the "gut level" to the sublimely spiritual. Therefore, the chakra system is a natural component of human-energy-field dynamics. In this system, there are seven major chakras as well as several secondary chakras. Two of these secondary chakras overlie the depressions in the palms of your hands. Most of us are unaware of their functioning. However, you can become sensitive to them with a little practice.

Experiential Exercise 3 will give you a "feel" for the singular characteristics of the human energy field. It is based on an ancient exercise that was used for different purposes. However, I like it because it will quickly give you an accurate idea of what the human energy field will feel like to you when you are doing the assessment phase of Therapeutic Touch.

EXPERIENTIAL EXERCISE 3

Feeling the Human Energy Field

1. Begin by quietly centering your consciousness.

2. Sit or stand in a comfortable position, and then place your hands so that your palms face each other.

3. Bring the palms of your hands together, but do not let them touch each other. About one-eighth to one-quarter of an inch should separate them.

4. Now separate your hands until they are about four inches apart. Then, in a slow, continuous motion, bring both hands together until they are again only slightly apart, as in their original position.

5. Once again separate your hands, this time drawing them apart about six inches. Then slowly bring them together until they are again one-eighth to one-quarter of an inch apart.

6. Separate your hands a final time so that they are approximately eight inches apart. This time, as you slowly bring them back to their original position, make slight, bouncy, lateral movements with your hands so that they move toward each other one or two inches at a time. As you are doing this, stay aware of any sensations you feel in your hands until they are once again about one-eighth to one-quarter of an inch apart.

7. Write down on a piece of paper your descriptions of what you felt during these bouncy movements.

It is interesting to do this exercise with other persons, either at the same time or at other times, and to compare your experiences. Try this exercise several times, remembering to begin by centering your consciousness. This exercise should not produce stress. To assure this, keep your wrists loose. There should be only minimal tension in your shoulder muscles as you hold up your hands, and you should be breathing naturally. Sweat will get you nowhere. It is your mind that you are using in this exercise. "Listen," that is, pay attention to your hands!

Most people have no difficulty in perceiving a sense of energy flow between their hands during this exercise. However, should you be one of the very few who do not sense anything distinctive, check that your attention is truly focused on the exercise and that you are maintaining an attitude of nonjudgmental inquiry into the nature of human energy flow. Sometimes you can increase your sensitivity to the energy by doing this exercise while having a living animal (cats respond very well) or plant or several fresh bean sprouts as the focus for your hand chakras. Living currents of energy flow have distinctive characteristics that nevertheless are quite subtle. Although they are present around us all the time, our Western culture does not recognize them and they are rarely brought to our attention. To overcome this handicap, you must be willing to invest adequate time and attention to become aware of a state of consciousness that, in the usual daily activities of living in our culture, is considered to be non-ordinary. This sensitization process is similar to training your ear to catch the nuances of interesting but foreign music or languages.

Comments on Exercise 3

With a little practice, the cues you pick up doing Experiential Exercise 3 will be quite specific. Mary Ann T., a former student, wrote the following in her journal:

> *February 14, 9 a.m.:* AH-HA! I've tried the self-knowledge test with the hands and *I did feel something!* It was

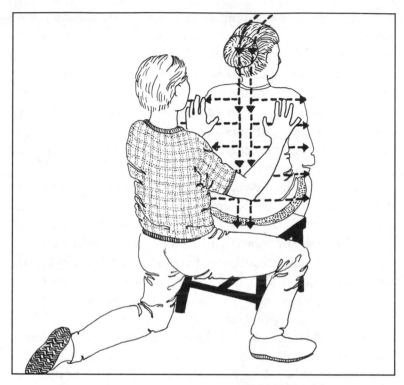

FIGURE 3. Assessing the

slightly different as I learned to "listen" more carefully. The sensations that I felt were heat, tingling, a sensation of pressure, and elasticity, so that the area between my hands felt like warm Jell-O or warm foam.

Another student, Jane, wrote:

> In doing the exercise of the hand energy centers, I found that I experienced more bounciness when my fingers were slightly separated. Also, I felt more changes in the field as I moved my hands apart. However, when my fingers were touching each other, the sensations of heat were more apparent. It is interesting that even though my hands are cold (I am working in my study), I distinctly felt heat—not warm hands—heat between my hands.

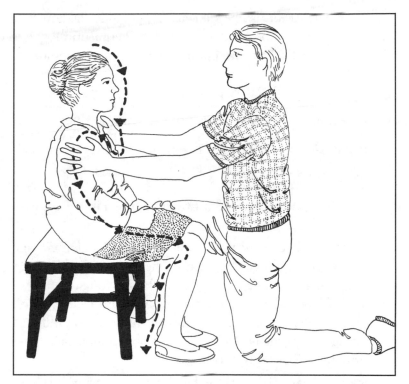

Healee's Energy Field

Experiential Exercise 3 is a simple and effective exercise from which it is possible to learn several things. It is a useful way to sense how the energy centers in the hands distinguish the various characteristics of the human energy field. It also exercises those centers so that they become more sensitive. In addition, the decided concentration you need to set up the field between your hands, and the shift in perception that occurs as you become more attentive to the subtleties of the field itself, can teach you how to stay on center. In fact, many people use this exercise as an occasion to practice centering.

The Assessment Technique

Therapeutic Touch is a natural potential. Therefore, you will find that you develop your own personal style of doing it. However, it is suggested that you use the following simple and reliable method several times in your beginning practice of Therapeutic Touch so that you have a background upon which to judge innovations.

EXPERIENTIAL EXERCISE 4

Basic Technique for Assessment of the Human Energy Field

In the assessment phase of Therapeutic Touch practice, begin by centering, as described above. Then:

1. Seat the healee or have him or her lie down in a comfortable position.

2. Stand at either the healee's front or back. (It is immaterial which you begin with.) Using the healee's spinal column as a visual reference, that is, as the body's longitudinal axis of bilateral symmetry, place your hands near the top of the healee's head. The palms of your hands should be facing toward the healee and about two to three inches from his or her body. (See figure 3.)

3. Starting near the top of the head, bring your hands slowly but steadily down through the healee's energy field. Gently sweep through the field, beginning with both hands near the healee's spinal column. Then sweep both hands in unison laterally, toward the periphery of the energy field, and back again to the spinal column.

4. Proceed level by level down toward the healee's feet. Do not stay in any place too long. Continue to sweep the field slowly but steadily, "listening" (acutely paying attention) to whatever cues your hand chakras are picking up.

5. Even if you are attracted to or concerned about a particular area, do not stop until you assess the healee's entire energy field. It is important at this time that you get a sense of the healee as a totality, as a unique being. After you have made your first assessment, go back over the

energy field and recheck the details that concern you, if it is still necessary at that time.

6. As your hands move down the field, keenly notice any differences you may feel between your hands, constantly comparing what you feel in one hand to what you feel in the other. If you do feel something on one side of the energy field that you don't feel on the other side, store in your mind what the sensation feels like to you and continue your rhythmic sweep of the field until you get down to the healee's feet.

7. Now go back to the opposite side of the body (the front or back, depending upon which side you have already done) and scan the energy field on that side of the body in the same fashion.

Note: The time it takes to assess one side of the energy field should be about thirty seconds. This is a new way of perceiving for you, so practice this exercise frequently.

Comments on Exercise 4

As you learn to "listen" attentively with the chakras in your hands, you will pick up messages or cues in subtle ways. Cues may come through many avenues of your sensorium: as vague hunches, passing impressions, flights of fancy, or, in precious moments, true insights or intuitions. Very frequently, the cues constellate into a clear visualization within your mind of an ongoing process or some aspect of it. Accept whatever impressions arise, and tuck them in the back of your mind without interrupting your assessment process. Continue until you feel that your evaluation is complete and you are ready to go on to the next stage of Therapeutic Touch.

An important part of this assessment process is testing your impressions against reality. If the healee improves or your impressions are proved correct in some other way, then you know you can rely on your mode of evaluation. At some later point in time, try to recapture your assessment experience and get a clear sense of how you tuned in to the cues. Obviously, if the messages from your senses turn out not to ring true in a reality test, search within yourself for another avenue of perception that may be more sensitive to a healee's condition.

Under any circumstances, and particularly while you are learning Therapeutic Touch, the key to eventual success is always to return to that centering place within yourself. It is this place that is the learning and testing ground for your growing understanding of the many facets of your consciousness. Use a journal to record your impressions over time, so that when you have a moment to sit down and review your material, you will have enough data upon which to make a considered judgment. Frequent practice is the best way to improve your skills, and you must provide yourself ample opportunity for this practice.

Recognizing Cues in the Healee's Energy Field

The "differences" you feel between your hands as you move down the healee's energy field can be quite explicit, and you will quickly learn to recognize them. These "differences" are actually cues to the states or conditions of various areas of the healee's energy field. You may notice a few peculiarities about your observations. One is that you do not feel the cues with the cutaneous, or surface tissues of your hands, but with the deep underlying tissues of your hands. For instance, if you feel heat as you scan the healee's energy field, it does not resemble the heat you feel if you put your hands on a hot stove. Rather, you feel the heat in the interior, deep tissues of your hands.

Another peculiarity involves the perceived temperature itself. The skin temperatures in the areas over which healers have felt heat during Therapeutic Touch assessments have been measured by sensitive thermocouples. However, there has never been an increase in the recorded skin temperature correlated with the heat perceived by the healers. Stranger yet is that in these studies the healers' hands themselves remained cool both to the touch and by measurement, even though the healers were picking up heat from the healees' energy fields. Obviously, Therapeutic Touch deals with a very different aspect or conception of temperature differential than the one we currently understand in biophysics. A more specific conclusion must await a different caliber of insightful studies.

As you become more practiced in the assessment phase of Therapeutic Touch, you may relate to at least five different levels of consciousness. These are all subjective states and, since there have been no significant research findings or in-depth studies on these states, they can be discussed only from an experiential perspective.

As a background against which to evaluate the different reality of cues sensed in the energy field, somewhat arbitrarily I have assigned the five levels of consciousness to the five major messages or cues that have been most commonly experienced by healers during Therapeutic Touch assessment. These data have been reported consistently since Dora Kunz and I began the development of Therapeutic Touch in 1972.

1. One level of consciousness involves the awareness of cues concerned with temperature differential, that is, sensations of heat, coldness, or the still coolness of a vacuum. These temperature differentials are the cues most frequently sensed.

2. Another level involves the magnetic drawing of the hand to a specific area of the healee's energy field. At this level of consciousness, congestion, pressure, or fullness may be perceived also.

3. A third level of consciousness involves cues described as "tinglings," "burstings of little bubbles," "pins and needles," or "little electric shocks."

4. A separate, fourth level of consciousness involves cues perceived as rhythmic pulsations in the healee's energy field.

5. A fifth level of consciousness is reserved for those insights into the healee's condition that are truly intuitive. At this level, cues are projected to the healer's consciousness in a manner that the healer may or may not be aware of. They "are just there" as information and need to be tested for reliability.

EXPERIENTIAL EXERCISE 5

The Emperor's Clothes

This exercise, "The Emperor's Clothes," is designed to test your perception of cues in the healee's energy field. I call the human energy field "the Emperor's Clothes" because, like the emperor's new clothes in the fairy tale of that name, the human energy field is invisible. To a bystander, the healer doing a Therapeutic Touch assessment seems to be attending to something that is invisible or imaginary.

Materials

A plastic bag, approximately ten inches wide by twelve inches long, and a pair of scissors.

Procedure

As in figure 4, cut one side of the plastic bag along dotted line A—B, so it can be laid open. Then cut along dotted line C—D so there is a hole in the corner of the plastic bag. Now put one arm of the healee through this hole in the plastic bag. The healee wears the Emperor's Clothes like a vest that has been cut in half.

To practice Therapeutic Touch assessment, engage the aid of another person willing to play the role of healee while you play the role of healer.

1. Give the Emperor's Clothes to this other person and, standing about eight to ten inches away from him or her, close your eyes.

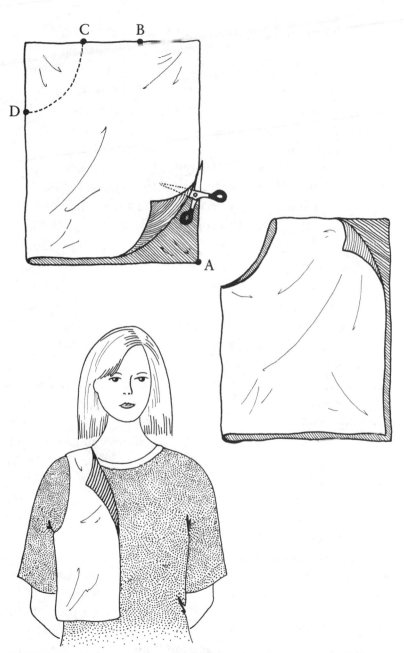

FIGURE 4. How to Make the Emperor's Clothes

2. With your eyes closed, have the healee put the Emperor's Clothes either over his or her right side, as shown in figure 4, or over his or her left side, by turning the vest inside out. The healee makes this choice without telling you.

3. Many years ago, Dora Kunz sensitively observed that the energy-field flow is dampened by materials such as the plastic bag that the healee is now wearing. Therefore, the two sides of the healee's energy field will not feel the same when you do your assessment. Without opening your eyes, reach out in the direction of the healee and do a Therapeutic Touch assessment of his or her energy field.

4. With your eyes shut, attempt to discern the "differences" that will tell you on which side of the healee's body the Emperor's Clothes are located.

5. Once you have made your decision, open your eyes and confirm your choice. It is fun now to change roles and find out how the other person does in the role of the healer.

Comments on Exercise 5

In all your work with Therapeutic Touch, maintain an inquiring mind. In actual practice, the key to helping the healee lies in the subtle cues you pick up in the patterns of energy flow of the healee's field. These patterns of energy are not composed of matter as we usually understand it; therefore, they may not be readily perceived by the simple physical senses, if at all. To become aware of them demands a different level of sensitivity, so you must be willing to explore beyond the gross senses with which you may be most familiar. This necessitates going within yourself while you are centered and seeking out the aspects of your consciousness that are responsive to the fine energies you encounter in the Therapeutic Touch interaction. This turning of your attention inward will reveal another, deeper level of awareness that in common daily activities is too often ignored or kept under tight control in our society.

To get beyond the rigid bonds of this control, I suggest that you identify with the cues you pick up; get all the information you can out of them. It may be useful to match your own breathing with the respiratory rate of the healee as you "reach out" with your energy field to assess his or her condition. Although you should sharply discipline any tendency you may have to fantasize, be sensitive to associative ideas that may well up in you as you assess the healee's energy field and thoughtfully evaluate their relevance.

However, also be willing to objectively test your impressions. Keep a journal of your Therapeutic Touch activities. An excellent way to teach yourself is to riffle through its pages at a later date, particularly if you are able to keep a verbatim account of your therapeutic interactions with your clients.

Consider the inferences and implications you impute to the cues you gather from the healee's energy field. Test your assumptions against laboratory reports, x-rays, other medical imageries, and technical reports, if they are available. Be impersonal in seeking out these findings. In using Therapeutic Touch, you are trying to help someone who is ill, not seeking justification that you are right. You are intervening in someone else's life, and you need to look for objective means of assuring yourself that the process you are using is useful to the situation.

Take every opportunity to become sensitive to the living energy field. If you are unable to work on people under your present circumstances, assess the energy fields of your pets or other domestic animals, the trees in your neighborhood (particularly if they are coniferous or eucalyptus trees, which radiate an immense energy field relative to their size), or groups of flowers. If you are pregnant—whether you are the mother or the father—gently assess the energy field of your growing baby as it comes to term. Many of my students have kept journals of such intimate interactions and shared their impressions within the family.

Another kind of sharing can occur when you do an assessment with a partner. Each of you completely assesses one side of the healee's energy field, then you switch positions and each assesses the other side. At the end, you compare notes and, on the basis of the ensuing discussion, decide together on the appropriate treatment of the healee. Such facets of Therapeutic Touch treatment will be discussed later in the book.

Assessing the Healee's Energy Field for Emotional Content

Assessment in Therapeutic Touch entails a different kind of intelligence than the kind you use in your casual affairs. It can, for instance, involve other ways of communicating that include still poorly understood functions of the psyche. With practice, you can learn to pick up sophisticated cues concerning the healee's emotional state. The following exercise, "Sensing the Emotions," is one that I developed specifically to enhance this aspect of Therapeutic Touch.

EXPERIENTIAL EXERCISE 6

Sensing the Emotions

This exercise is most challenging when it is done with several people who have a common understanding of Therapeutic Touch and who accept emotions as a form of human energy. However, all people can do this exercise, whatever their background. Except when severely repressed, all people portray emotions vividly and freely that are easily conveyed and quickly picked up by other persons.

Materials

Several slips of paper, one for each person in the group, and a pen or pencil.

Procedure

Begin by copying onto each slip of paper one of the following emotions and its synonyms:

AGITATION
irritability edginess exasperation

ANGER
infuriation enragement resentfulness

ANXIETY
apprehension foreboding euphoria

APATHY
indifference unresponsiveness lack of feeling

CARING
concern love protectiveness

DEPRESSION
melancholy despair despondency

FEAR
terror dread panic

GRIEF
sorrow remorse anguish

HOPE
trust expectation anticipation

HOPELESSNESS
futility impossibility unattainability

JOY
jubilance exultation delight

LONELINESS
separation friendlessness solitude

PAIN
agony discomfort hurt

VIBRANT HEALTH
vigor vitality vivaciousness

1. Each person takes one slip of paper. Nobody but the holder sees what is written on it.

2. Next, each person pairs off with a partner. Preferably the partners are not well known to each other.

3. Each pair of partners then decides which one of them will be the sender and which will be the receiver for this exercise. The sender then sits in a chair, and the receiver stands directly behind the chair. Both persons should have a notepad and pen or pencil nearby.

4. If you are the sender, begin by quietly centering. When you feel on center, go back in your memory to a time when you were gripped by the emotion noted on your piece of paper. Clearly visualize that experience and actually feel the body tones and mood you felt then. Be there, at that time and in that space. Live that experience once again.

   In the event that you cannot bring yourself to relate to that emotion, choose another slip of paper.

   If you are willing to recapture the experience, but you do not think you are adequately expressing the emotion, stay on center and silently say the words on the paper over and over to yourself, or clearly visualize the words in your mind.

   Nod your head as a signal to your partner when you feel in the throes of the appropriate emotion.

5. If you are the receiver, stand in a relaxed position and quietly center yourself. When you have received the signal from your partner, place your hand just above either of his or her shoulders so that there is a space of two to three inches between your hand and the shoulder.

   From the moment that your hand comes into the range of the sender's energy field, be open and aware of any imagery that arises in your mind—pictures, colors, sounds, words, music, noises, tastes, smells, and so on. Store the memory of these first images in the back of your mind, and then allow other secondary images to arise. However, do not force or structure them; merely let them flow by your mind's eye. After two to three minutes, jot down your memories of the images in your notebook, as well as any associative words or thoughts that well up in your consciousness.

6. At the end of this interaction, the sender, who has remained on center during this time, now also writes down any aspects of the experience that seem significant, particularly any personal reactions to the receiver.

7. Do not speak to each other about your experiences at this time. First, change roles and repeat the process. After you have been both sender and receiver, compare both experiences with your partner.

Comments on Exercise 6

This exercise offers some insight into how to use the Therapeutic Touch assessment for becoming sensitive to any emotional overlay of the healee's problems. A variation of this exercise involves having the person who is playing the role of sender choose one of a limited range of colors—for instance, blue, yellow, or green—without telling the receiver which color he or she has chosen. The sender then clearly visualizes the color, perhaps as the blue of the sky, or the yellow glint of the sun, or the green of grass, or whatever best expresses the color in mind. The receiver then centers, does a Therapeutic Touch assessment, and tries to determine the chosen color.

In-Depth Assessment of the Human Energy Field

You will be able to assess problems of increasing depth as you build up a body of knowledge about the Therapeutic Touch process and use it with confidence. You will also develop a repertoire of skills based on your own personal experiences, and you may discover a growing sensitivity in yourself that goes beyond, or in a different direction from, more formal diagnostic methods.

An example of this is described in a letter from another former student, Kim, who works with nonverbal children on a pediatric surgical service in Minnesota. Her letter report tells me that she has uncovered previously unknown abscesses and subluxations in these children during her use of the Therapeutic Touch assessment.

As another example, I have a package of laboratory reports and neurological consultations from a large medical center in Massachusetts. The woman whom these reports concern had been diagnosed as having Parkinson's syndrome, and she had come to me for Therapeutic Touch. Shortly before receiving this package, I had been requested to see a woman with complex brain injuries that had resulted in Parkinson-like symptoms. This first woman had responded surprisingly well to Therapeutic Touch within a very short time. The memory of this first woman's energy field and response to treatment was very much with me when I saw the second woman.

After doing a thorough assessment of the second woman, I did not conclude that she had Parkinson's syndrome. After careful deliberation, I told her of my reservations and recommended that she get a second neurological opinion. She followed my suggestion and sought out another neurologist. The parcel of reports are from the analysis of that second examination, and it confirms my own assessment. The cover letter from the attending physician says, in part, "The main issue is whether you have Parkinson's syndrome, and Dr. ─────── does not feel that you do, and he has given a very detailed schedule of how to cut back on the medication."

An excerpt, in some detail, from another student's journal gives a sense of how personal skills might be used in practice. Sonia had just returned to class after being treated for an ectopic pregnancy. She wrote the following account:

After all the students had left the room, I asked Dr. Krieger for a Therapeutic Touch assessment. I told her that I was not feeling well and needed her help. She placed her hand over my head and immediately told me that something was really quite wrong. She said that I was very anxious, which I realized was true but nevertheless wondered at her continuing concern as she went on with the assessment.

She quietly talked to me while raising her hand up and bringing it down briskly several times along the sides of my body. She then advised me to go home and to go to bed immediately when I got there and said that I should phone my doctor. I sensed the urgency in her voice. She even offered to drive me home, but I told her that I had another class following hers. She advised me to skip the class and go straight home. She even went with me to my statistics lab and waited for me while I wrote a note to the professor.

I was still astounded at what Dr. Krieger had told me, so I asked her what she had "felt" as we walked to the elevator. Aside from a vague pain in my lower abdomen, I truly felt capable of walking. I really didn't feel bad enough to warrant going home immediately and so on. Dr. Krieger said that the acute problem was localized in my lower abdomen, but her greater concern was that the problem was now becoming systemic to the point of considerable seriousness. She had also felt that I was not stable yet, and that I had significant amounts of fluid in my lungs.

I telephoned my husband, who was still at work, and Dr. Krieger stayed with me the whole time that I waited for him to drive to the university. She even went out into that howling snowstorm to buy me a cup of mint herbal tea. While waiting for her to return with the tea, I stood near a radiator in the corridor and did some relaxation exercises she had taught me, and then I also did some Therapeutic Touch to myself.

I thought about what Dr. Krieger had found out about my condition and, frankly, wondered what she might be doing to the tea she was bringing back to me. At the time, I did not think that what was going on in my mind about Dr. Krieger was funny at all. I simply felt relieved and very grateful for what she was doing for me, and I knew that I would welcome whatever else she wanted to do to help me.

When she returned, the warmth of the tea made me feel better, and we quietly talked, while other students on their way to class streamed around us, until my husband arrived. He had seen Dr. Krieger on a television program a few nights before and took her words seriously as she quickly reviewed what had gone on. We all went out into that snowy night, and my husband and I went straight home.

Less than an hour after we reached home, I experienced severe pain in my abdomen. My husband rushed me to the hospital. Blood tests were done, which revealed an abnormally high white-blood cell count that indicated a severe infection. Chest x-rays were taken, and they demonstrated a right-sided pleural effusion—fluid in the lungs. Sonograms revealed further fluid accumulations in my abdomen, and there was indication I might have another ectopic pregnancy. The doctor decided to admit me to the hospital immediately.

In practice, what you pick up first in the Therapeutic Touch assessment is often relative to the superficial condition of the healee. I find it useful to maintain an attitude of searching inquiry. "What else?" is the question I put before myself as I scan the healee's energy field. I have coined a term out of necessity to indicate a human ultrasensorial dimension that transcends or goes beyond the three physical dimensions of length, width, and breadth. It comes into play when you are doing advanced practices of Therapeutic Touch. The term is *inth,* and it is fairly descriptive of where you "go" during the experience of journeying inside yourself. After I've asked myself, what else? I plunge more deeply into the therapeutic interaction with the healee, always using as a background what I know to be my most *inth* level of consciousness, and keeping on center, of course.

As the healer-healee interaction deepens, the energy fields of both parties seem to mesh so that it is easier for the healer to identify or empathize with the healee. A kind of resonance occurs between them, enabling the healer to get a clearer idea of the healee's condition. The caution here is that you must take care to monitor yourself against impulsive thinking, wishful thinking, or fantasy. Make very sure that you are responding to real or actual cues, and take every precaution to rule out figments of your imagination. You have undertaken the role of healer; keep in mind your responsibility to give the healee a fair representation of your abilities.

Keep a journal or some other record of your Therapeutic Touch assessments. In reviewing it from time to time, note the similarities and differences in the various patterns of energy you cue into as you assess healees with a variety of problems. Such a record is an excellent learning tool. Compare your notes with those of others who are practicing Therapeutic Touch. Organize a support system among practitioners in your vicinity and use the telephone, computer electronic bulletin board, or fax machine to compare notes or make referrals.

Most importantly, whenever the opportunity is available, check your Therapeutic Touch assessments against objective evidence about the healee under consideration. Bring to each experience in the Therapeutic Touch process everything you have previously experienced and everything you have learned that might be useful. In summary, be totally present for the healee.

Chapter 3

HOW HUMAN ENERGIES
ARE USED FOR HEALING

In general, healing involves the conscious, full engagement of the healer's own energies in the compassionate interest of helping another person. In this sense, the healer can be considered a human support system. There are a few prerequisites. Among the most important is that the healer should have a strong motivation to help or heal—a compassionate need to heal—and the intentionality to see this come about. The term *intentionality* implies that the healer has not only the will but also a specific goal in mind. That is, the healer understands how to facilitate the healing of a particular person.

There are also prerequisites regarding the healee. The healee must have a willingness to change and an acceptance of change (from the state of being ill). This may sound strange, since one would think that every sick person would want to put illness and weakness and perhaps pain out of his or her life. However, it is sometimes the case that there are secondary gains to be had by being incapacitated and therefore having society's permission to be dependent on others.

To heal another person, in one sense the healer interposes his or her own energy field between the healee and the illness. From another point of view, however, the healer sensitively draws upon the universal energies that are the backdrop to all living events and within which both healer and healee are figures sharing a unitary nature.[1] Energy fields are nonmaterial; nevertheless, you do have physical access to them. This is readily understandable if you recognize that human emotions are a form of human energy.

Emotions have gross physiological effects that range from the subtle electrical charges that conduct primitive emotions through the deep neural recesses of the brain's limbic system to more obvious effects such as sweat on bare skin in testimonial to fear or other strong passions. Moreover, the physical structure itself can be destroyed by uncontrolled emotions. A case in point would be a peptic ulceration following prolonged anxiety.

In Therapeutic Touch, the assessment process is a direct experience of another's energy field. As demonstrated in Experiential Exercise 6, through this sensitive interaction you as the assessor can pick up cues that indicate emotional as well as physical problems of the healee. By the end of the assessment, it would also be useful for you to have specific thoughts on what could be done to help the healee and why you would be doing it. Most frequently, the cues you pick up in the healee's energy field during the assessment are one or a combination of the following:

- Temperature differentials, such as a sense of heat or cold.
- Pressure, or feelings of congestion in the energy flow.
- Changes in or lack of synchronization in the intrinsic rhythmicity of the healee's energy field.
- Localized weak electric shocks or tingly feelings as you move the energy centers in the palms of your hands through the healee's energy field.

How can these simple, subjective impressions be translated into an effective healing technique? The answer lies in a principle that is perhaps unbelievable to persons brought up solely within the perspective of Western culture, but which is used throughout the world by people of other cultures. This is the simple principle of opposites in the treatment of illness. Underlying this principle of opposites is the concept of health as a state in which the body's energies are in balance.

When a person's energies are out of balance, the person becomes ill. Therefore, it is the healer's charge to rebalance the healee's energies. For instance, among the Latinos of Central America who treat illnesses nutritionally, if a *curandero* determines that the patient has what would be considered to be a "cold" illness, that patient would be treated with "hot" foods. The opposite would be true in the case of a "hot" illness.

A somewhat similar rationale underlies Therapeutic Touch, except that the concept of balancing refers directly to human energy systems. Within this context, if you as the healer pick up cues of heat in the healee's energy field, you would act to "cool" that area of the field. This can be done in several ways. One of the most direct and simple is to first take a moment to clearly remember what it feels like to be cold. Actually imagine yourself being cold by replicating the memory of a cool feeling throughout your own energy field. The effect is somewhat analogous to clearly recalling a happy incident and then feeling light and joyous in memory of the occasion. In this case, you actually feel cold by reenacting your reaction to the nip of chilliness.

Once that occurs, you consciously focus and project that sense of cold through the energy centers of your hands (in the energy field overlying your palms) to the area of the healee's energy field where you picked up the cue of heat. When you project this sense of coolness, do not allow yourself to "push" the cold energies; there is no need for that. Simply concentrate on remembering with clarity what cold feels like, and then effortlessly project that distinct mind picture through your hand energy centers to the healee's energy field. Permit your mind to work for you and to follow your intentionality.

Other cues would be balanced in a more physical manner. For instance, if you felt pressure in the healee's energy field during the assessment, you would attempt to reduce that pressure. This can be done by moving (with the energy centers of your hands) the congested area of the healee's energy field toward the periphery of the field. This allows for a resumption of a more natural energy flow. If you felt an irregularity in the rhythmicity of the healee's energy flow, you would project energy of an even, synchronous nature.

If you felt little, weak "electric shocks," you would act to dampen them. If you felt a tingly sensation during the assessment, you would try to smoothe the energy so that there is a less irritated, more coherent energetic flow.

Although too little is understood about the underlying dynamics of human energy systems at this time to thoroughly understand why these cue-specific techniques work, the important fact is that they do indeed work. The healee feels better, the pain is relieved, and an incredibly fast relaxation response occurs. Invariably, the healee has a sense of well-being that persists long after the Therapeutic Touch practitioner has gone. Most importantly, healing is facilitated and in many cases accelerated.

Although human energies are nonmaterial, the physical body does register the effects of these invisible forces in its material structures, as in the case of the destruction of tissues in a peptic ulcer. You can physically perceive the nerve conduction of noxious stimuli instantaneously, as, for instance, when pain is reflected in a facial grimace, or when deep concern is heard in the voice, even if it is only conjured up in the mind as fantasy.

Emotions can also be conveyed to another person silently, through body language, and yet have a physical effect on the recipient. For example, a parent may be caught in the throes of some inner turmoil and may communicate anger by no more than a glance to a child who is nearby. As he or she catches the emotional impact of the parent's anger, the child may immediately react physiologically, even though the parent never physically touches the child. In fact, the memory of the incident and its repetitive recall could be enough to open the doors to future psychosomatic illness in the child.

However, in the case of such nonmaterial energies coming from invisible energy centers, how do you know with certainty—as an incontrovertible, perceptual "fact"—that an effect has been transmitted? Moreover, how do you rule out possible, though nonapparent, intervening factors that might harbor the actual cause of the effect? If firsthand experience can be a criterion for you, the following exercise will help you answer such questions for yourself. This exercise takes advantage of a long-known, but little-understood fact: human energies, such as those dealt with in Therapeutic Touch, can be directed intentionally into a wad of ordinary cotton batting. Cotton so treated will store the energy for a length of time, during which the energy can be felt by another person as a "fact."

EXPERIENTIAL EXERCISE 7

Directing Human Energy

Before beginning this exercise, it would be useful to review Experiential Exercise 6. A partner is needed for this exercise.

Materials

One piece of unsterilized, 100 percent cotton batting that has been cut into pieces approximately three inches by six inches for each person.

Procedure

1. Take a moment to center your consciousness.
2. When you feel centered, pick up your piece of cotton and place it on the open palm of one hand, letting it lie there loosely.
3. Place the palm of your other hand above the cotton pad, about two to four inches away from its surface.
4. Direct the flow of your energy downward, from the hand center above the cotton, through the cotton pad, and into the energy center of your lower hand holding the cotton pad. Since energy follows the line of focus of your attention, you can perform this part of the procedure most effectively by focusing your attention and clearly visualizing the energy flowing all the way through the cotton pad and then continuing into your underlying hand.

5. Continue to focus this flow for two to three minutes, being sensitive to any differences that you feel in the energy center of your underlying hand. Do not bring your upper hand into contact with the cotton; continue to hold it two to four inches above the pad.

6. When you perceive a difference in energy flow, exchange pads with another person doing this exercise and quickly assess the energy field of your partner's cotton pad. Almost immediately, you will become aware that your partner's cotton pad feels distinctly different from yours. Most often, this difference will feel like extreme heat.

7. Write down what you feel as you continue to assess your partner's cotton pad. When you and your partner are both done with your descriptions, compare your experiences. Invariably, you will find that your cotton also felt much hotter to your partner than his or her own.

8. Exchange opinions on why you think this happens and then change partners with another couple. Repeat the exercise with your new partner and see if the general rule holds.

———————————————————————————————————

This exercise brings home with special cogency the realization that Therapeutic Touch deals with the human energy field rather than only the physical body. In Therapeutic Touch, your attention is concentrated on interpenetrating the energy field of the healee, not on merely contacting the healee's skin. This energy field is not made of matter in its familiar sense, but instead uses energy to express its characteristics and attributes. Because of this, learning to pick up cues during the assessment phase of Therapeutic Touch is very important. In becoming sensitive to these cues, you can map out the energetic state of the healee. Then healing can occur through the appropriate direction, modulation, or guidance of energy using specific intention and clear visualization. The healing energy interpenetrates the affected tissues of the healee's body and works at its own level.

This is not a concept that is easy to understand, I realize. This fact was demonstrated to me in an amusing manner some years ago. I had been brought over from the U.S. mainland to Oahu, Hawaii, as a guest lecturer for the University of Hawaii. In the midst of a lecture on Therapeutic Touch, I realized that the idea of energy-field penetration was not coming across clearly. I stopped the lecture with the intention of finding out where the difficulty lay. After a bit of semantic confusion, we finally resorted to pidgin English and came up with a clarifying phrase that conveyed the idea graphically: *poka-tru*. To *poka tru* literally meant to "poke through" the energy field by visualizing the energy flow going through the more compacted matter of the physical body of the healee. I could not have wished for a more descriptive phrase!

For example, in Experiential Exercise 7, the temperature change you may have felt in the cotton occurred because the focused energy had *poka-tru*; that is, the energy flow penetrated through the matter of the cotton pad and changed the energy level of the cotton. However, to explain why you feel the temperature change more readily in the cotton pad of another person than in your own, I'd have to resort to mainland speculation.

I suggest that you not hesitate to learn from everything around you. There are many levels of energy associated with living systems, and plants and animals make very good test objects for learning to recognize the kinds of energies you can project. With rare exception, no harm will come to them; rather, they will benefit from your compassionate concern.

All domestic animals can be helped by Therapeutic Touch. Many persons have used it on their small pets, and several of "Krieger's Krazies" (people who have been taught Therapeutic Touch by me) have used it on their horses and cows. If you are sensitive to their special needs, many injured birds and wild animals can also be helped.

A particularly interesting exercise is to use Therapeutic Touch to assist in the healthy sprouting of seedlings and the recovery of unhealthy plants. I find that succulents such as aloe vera and cacti are especially responsive. One of my students, Linda, wrote in her journal about her experience with doing Therapeutic Touch to her plants:

> About six months ago a friend brought me a lovely hanging plant. I seem to kill all plants, and, sure enough, this plant was dying a slow and pitiful death in spite of my care and concern. Since all else had failed, recently I decided to try Therapeutic Touch on the plant. To be honest, I have been doing Therapeutic Touch faithfully, but I'm not really sure of what I feel. However, I'm sure that I do feel something. It's just "different'; I don't know how else to explain it. Well, the plant likes Therapeutic Touch. New shoots are coming up, the plant is perking up, and so am I! I think that my plant-healee will be a good teacher for me.

Putting the Treatment Together

Since your desire to help a healee arises out of compassion for his or her pain or illness, use everything at your command, all of your past experience and education, in the healee's interest. Start wherever you are. For instance, use observation: What does the healee's body language tell you? Does the posture tell you that there is a guarding or protecting of certain areas of the body? Look for signs of fatigue or strain, hyperactivity or scattered attention, distraction or restlessness. Have the healee be either seated comfortably or lying down. You as the healer need to stand or sit nearby while doing Therapeutic Touch so that you can easily see these subtle cues.

It is said in the literature that the major energy flows in a human being move from the crown of the head toward the feet.[2-4] Therefore, begin the appropriate therapeutic measures in the uppermost areas of the healee's energy field and then successively treat the lower areas. Remember that you are working with the healee's energy field.

Treat the healee by placing one hand in the healee's energy field over the area in which you sensed a cue during assessment. Place your other hand in the energy field on the opposite side of the healee, and then *poka-tru* the energy field as you did with the cotton in the exercise. If the opposite side is inaccessible (for example, if the healee is lying on that side), place your other hand anywhere in the healee's energy field; you are directing or modulating energy with the powers of your mind, and this is a nonphysical human-energy-field phenomenon that you are dealing with.

This treatment process is not quite as easy as it sounds, but your ability will improve as you practice and gain facility in concentration and focus. The general principle you are working with at this phase is rebalancing, which is done by projecting energy of a nature that is opposite to that of the cues you sensed in the assessment.

Move your hands in a rhythmical way at a moderate rate, treating the central areas of the healee's field and then working toward its periphery. Include areas of the field that are beyond and below the feet. Have as your intention any of the following ploys, although you need not limit yourself to these:

- The facilitation of energy flow
- The stimulation of energy flow
- The mobilization of congestion or pressure in the energy field
- The dampening or quieting of energetic activity
- The synchronization of rhythmicity in the energy flow

Do not perform any of these healing activities mechanically. Perform them as specific responses to the cues you picked up during the assessment, holding in mind the perspective of the healee as an integrated being.

In the assessment phase of Therapeutic Touch, you as the healer identify with the healee's energy field in order to pick up cues that might indicate energy imbalance. In the rebalancing phase, however, you use your own healthy self as a model for repat-terning the energies of the healee. This does not necessarily mean that you use only "personal" energies in the healing process. Rather, you use your efficient faculties for accessing the necessary energies, and you act as a human support system to help the healee to heal himself or herself.

Although Therapeutic Touch may not perform miracle cures, it has proven itself both safe and helpful in appropriate cases. It is only by working with Therapeutic Touch that you can get an adequate sense of its dynamics and thoughtfully appreciate and evaluate its worth.

Major Techniques of Therapeutic Touch

The techniques used in Therapeutic Touch are specific to the healee; however, there are three major techniques and several sub-sidiary ones. All of them begin with centering your consciousness and quietly relating to your inner state of being as described in chapter 2. This inner state of quietude allows you to shift your at-tention from the clamor of daily living that incessantly competes for notice to a more neutral place where you can consider the needs of another with equipoise and considered judgment. Centered, you can approach the problems of the healee with an open mind. The details of the problems will then have the opportunity to im-press themselves freshly on your consciousness.

The Conscious Direction of Human Energies

Of the three major techniques used by healers in Therapeutic Touch, only one, the direction of energy, has been mentioned so far. In this technique, energy follows the attention of your mind. At the same time, there is a complex focusing of your chakras, or energy centers, on the object of your attention. This will be dis-cussed in the next chapter. With self-discipline and focus, your mind can intentionally direct energies over quite long distances within your own body. During biofeedback exercises, this allows you to warm your hands or deliberately relax even under conditions of stress. A way to prove the ability of your mind to move energy with intention and without recourse to instrumentation is suggested in the next exercise.

EXPERIENTIAL EXERCISE 8

Directing Energy through the Healee

For the purposes of this experiential exercise, three people are needed. One person plays the role of healee, and the other two play the roles of healer A and healer B.

Procedure

1. The healee removes his or her shoes and sits crosswise on a chair so that his or her back is easily accessible to healer A (who stands behind the healee) and his/her feet are easily reached by healer B (who stands in front of the healee).

2. Healer A stands behind the healee so that one hand can be placed over each of the healee's kidneys. The kidneys are in the back, just above the hips and inside the lower ribcage. (See figure 5.)

3. Healer B either kneels or sits in a comfortable position at the healee's feet so that her or his hand chakras have access to the healee's foot chakras. These foot chakras, or energy centers, are located in the regions of the healee's energy field underlying the arches of the feet. (See figure 5.)

4. Both healers and the healee begin by centering—the healers so that they can be more keenly aware of the energy flow, and the healee to maintain balance while being sensitive to the dynamics of the interaction.

5. If you are healer A, attempt to send energy from your hand chakras, which are poised over the healee's kidneys, through the healee's energy field and out the healee's foot chakras. This direction of energy is done with your mind

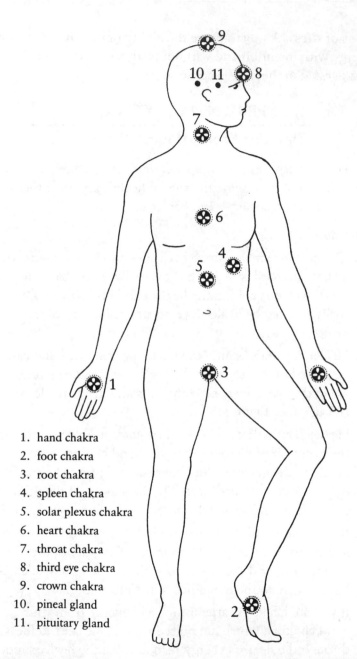

1. hand chakra
2. foot chakra
3. root chakra
4. spleen chakra
5. solar plexus chakra
6. heart chakra
7. throat chakra
8. third eye chakra
9. crown chakra
10. pineal gland
11. pituitary gland

FIGURE 5. Major Anatomical Sites Used in Therapeutic Touch

by firmly focusing your attention on the healee's feet and clearly visualizing the energy flowing from the kidney area to the feet. This energy flow can be aided by synchronizing your conscious direction with the exhalation of your breath. However, tension should not build up during this procedure. Simply allow the energy to flow naturally and without effort from your hand chakras to the healee's kidneys. Put your attention on the end result you wish to accomplish: the quickened flow of energy from the healee's kidneys to her or his foot energy centers.

6. Meanwhile, if you are healer B, focus your attention on assessing the healee's energy field in the region underlying his or her foot chakras. Of particular interest are any changes or differences in the frequency or intensity of energy flow that you may sense. The inference is that any changes in the energy flow are related to healer A's direc-

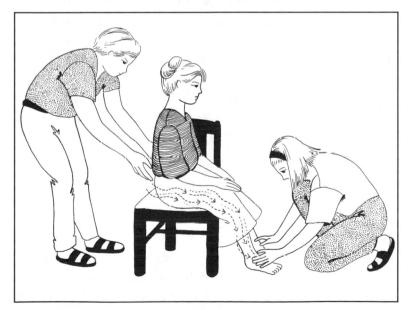

FIGURE 6. Directing Energy Through the Healee

tion of energy. This can be validated by having healer A stop directing energy for a few moments, during which time you reevaluate and compare the energy in the foot chakras.

7. After the quickened flow is verified by healer B, change roles with the other healer and repeat the exercise. Also, the healee can change roles with one of the healers and repeat the exercise. When each of you has had an opportunity to direct energy and have it verified, discuss your findings with each other.

Comments on Exercise 8

The kidney/adrenal areas of the human energy field are very safe sites from which to work. In the two decades that I have been using this exercise in my classes, there have never been any untoward reactions in persons playing any of the roles. In clinical situations, it seems that the kidney/adrenal sites are extremely efficient in drawing upon the kind of energies used in Therapeutic Touch. The patient feels vivified afterward, and even novice healers can feel distinct sensations when their hand energy centers are placed over the kidney areas on an ill person. Because these sites are so safe and effective, a general Therapeutic Touch practice has developed to treat these sites, particularly in cases of fatigue or exhaustion.

As in other health practices, you continually learn from experience. For instance, you can easily find distinctive signals of tension and fatigue in the energy field overlying the nuchal muscles, in the back of the neck. You can interface Therapeutic Touch techniques with shiatsu, acupressure, or massage for this problem.

Therapeutic Touch in the energy field over the heart frequently conveys a sense of deep caring to the healee. This creates a sedative effect and induces a consequent relaxation response. Because of this, it is a site often used by nurses, anesthesiologists, doctors, and other health practitioners, particularly before hospital procedures about which the patient might be apprehensive. The simple placement of a hand over a person's heart can also be used in a most beautiful manner in hospices to ease a person's final transition. This can be done by staff or volunteers who have been especially taught or by relatives who might like to share the last moments with those they love. Many other Therapeutic Touch techniques are discussed in chapter 5.

However, there are some situations in which Therapeutic Touch is either not done or done only in a very limited way. The possible effects of Therapeutic Touch are not adequately understood in these situations, and it makes good sense to exercise intelligent caution with them. One such instance concerns working in the energy field directly over a person's head in the case of cranial injuries. You should also be cautious not to work too energetically with near-term pregnant women. In both of these cases, the possible energetic complexities that might be involved with intervention are not fully understood. Therefore, if it is felt that Therapeutic Touch might be beneficial, the techniques need to be used sensitively, gently, and for a very short time—not more than two minutes in any one session. You can always come back at a later time, check on the progress of the healee and, if it is warranted, again use Therapeutic Touch.

As a practitioner of Therapeutic Touch, never tense up and "push" energy in an exertive manner. Never sweat. Energy flow is natural and, as noted above, its direction originates in the mind as an effortless, nonphysical, therapeutic employment of the self. In many cases of a serious nature, and with babies, there is a noticeably better effect when Therapeutic Touch is used sensitively and gently for short periods. With acute or traumatic cases, this is particularly a good general rule, for you can come back and do other sessions at a later time. Meanwhile, the interim can serve as an opportunity to observe the effects on the healee.

Equally obvious is another rule of thumb: If you don't know, don't do. As a therapist, you must use Therapeutic Touch in a conscious manner. This means that you need to know (from the assessment phase) where the problem lies in the healee's energy field, what therapeutic ploy to use, and why you are to do a given technique. Less than this may constitute irresponsible intervention. In cases where you do not know what to do, refer the healee to an appropriate person who can help.

Modulating Human Energies

When assessing certain healees during Therapeutic Touch practice, you may realize that the problem is not so much the depletion of energies as the redistribution of them. Toning up or toning down the quality or intensity of energy states may be needed. At these times, modulation or regulation of energy flow is useful.

One very good, natural way of modulating energy flow is to visualize colors as you project energy to the healee. How color modulates energy is little understood. However, it seems reasonable to assume that the transaction occurs in an analogous way to the voice being modulated to convey emotional content or underline meaning.

Like a sound, a color is a wavelength of energy, the specific wavelength depending upon the specific color. Repeated clinical tests with Therapeutic Touch have shown that visualization of a specific color has a specific effect. For instance, in the case of hyperactivity, visualization by a healer of a calm, cool color such as a clear royal blue serves to calm the healee. In my personal repertoire of techniques, I do not envision the royal blue like a solid pigment on an artist's palette but as a clear light of that particular hue.

The choices of colors to use in specific circumstances comes from a series of studies performed several years ago under the direction of Dora Kunz, who has provided a special, keen insight to the development of Therapeutic Touch over the years. In these studies, stage lights with gelatin slides of various colors were used as models for the visualization of the colors. After experiencing particular colors, subjects would try to clearly visualize those colors and then project the quality of their experiences to volunteers with various illnesses. Formal records were kept of the studies, which were especially successful with people who had hypertension and upon whom subjects projected the color of royal blue. In controlled trials, both the systolic and the diastolic blood-pressure readings went down significantly.

Over time, a wide range of colors proved useful for other conditions. The clear royal blue was highly reliable, and its use was generalized to all conditions requiring a sedative effect. A vibrant yellow light was stimulating to healees, and green had a neutral but energizing effect.

Curious about these results, for many years I have studied the use of colors in cultures around the world. I have found a strong correlation in the way these same three colors are used in art, decoration, and the creation of religious objects.

I get a workable appreciation of the energetic value of a color by sitting in the colored light cast by the sun as its rays beam through a stained-glass window. For me, the blue light cast through a stained-glass depiction of the Mother of the World conveys a distinctive sense of calmness and serenity. It is this specific blue that I recall to mind when I am working with someone who is in a high energy state that is out of control, such as panic, fear, or acute anxiety. I simulate this blue's characteristic rhythm and flow within myself. I also use it with physical problems that involve inflammation of tissues, with elevated temperatures, and, as noted above, with hypertension. Importantly, projecting this particular blue also facilitates a relaxation response in the healee.

For no rational reason that I can pinpoint, a shade of yellow-gold resembling the glints of sunshine on moving wavelets of a summer sea works best as a visualization when I want to stimulate or energize someone's energy field.

My choice for a mind model of neutral green is as utilitarian as the object itself is ubiquitous: a meadow of green grass. I use this green to find within myself a "vibe" or wavelength of energy that reflects a gentle yet vibrant sense of the fine balance characterizing a healing milieu.

ing that these three colors can reliably cover such situations, but extensive experience over the past ndicates that this is so. I suspect that when a person color, it is his or her reflected body tone that transmits the sen.. color and gives it meaning. You can experience this by walking outdoors under a green canopy of leaves and feeling a sense of well-being.

As in all techniques of Therapeutic Touch, expertise depends on experiential knowledge that has been tested against objective evidence. Although blue, yellow, and green serve for most occasions, you may find over time that other colors (that are specific wavelengths of energy) are appropriate for various situations. For instance, you might find that a rose color seems right when dealing with frightened children, or when you want to express compassionate concern or love. The possibilities for healing with color are considerable, and most probably colors will arise in your consciousness as the occasion demands. Modulation of energies in yourself goes on naturally and constantly in response to your everyday experiences. The implicit charge, however, when you project energy onto another person is to be consciously and responsibly aware of the subtle effects of this interaction.

Experiential Exercise 9 is a guided imagery to assist you in gaining a sense of what the modulation of energy with color feels like.

EXPERIENTIAL EXERCISE 9

Appreciating the Energetic Characteristics of Color

Please refer to Experiential Exercise 2 for suggestions on guided imagery practice. This guided imagery explores the energetic characteristics of the colors blue, yellow, and green. Begin by sitting or lying in a comfortable position, gentling your breath, and closing your eyes.

You have come with me to Montana, "the last best place." As you step out of our vehicle, you look up and know why it is called Big Sky Country. The sky is an overarching vault of clear, depthless royal blue that reaches to the horizons of space, and you feel its unlimited sense of serenity. You are at peace with yourself as you drink in the unbroken stillness that radiates from this undisturbed, calm blue quietude.

You are relaxed and at ease with the gentle blue energy. You feel mellow and understood. As though you are in a state of grace, you feel surrounded by a deep, caring sense of tender compassion that comprehends and values who you really are. You feel profoundly touched by this personal recognition and, for a moment, feel at one with your innermost true self.

As you drink in the serenity of the sky, the golden sunlight pours down on you. Glinting pinpoints of fiery yellow sparks joyously dance as they stream toward you, and *through* you, in an endless flow. They are like white-gold energy packets of scintillating light that burst upon you like the effervescent bubbles in a newly opened bottle of champagne.

These sparks impart a sense of vibrant being. You feel a tingling ecstasy of aliveness. Their radiance bathes you in a focused shower of powerful life-energy forces that quickens and stimulates your awareness of the exquisite beauties as well as the formidable challenges of life. Your body feels warm and energized, invigorated and vitalized by the luminous, glowing flow of living energy.

Before you is a growth of trees, and you walk toward them. Their full, green branches arch in a translucent canopy above you as you enter the sylvan woods. The sunlight filters through the green foliage and, in its verdant shade, you feel comfortable—neither too hot nor too cold—without stress, and in balance with nature around

you. You are on center, and in a state of effortless
equipoise.

Now a slight refreshing breeze sweeps through the
depths of the forest of green light. Quietly take a deep
breath of the clean, fully oxygenated atmosphere that the
green grove freely discharges to you in return for the car-
bonous waste products you exhale and no longer need. As
the vitalizing breath fills your body, know that all in the
universe is in dynamic balance—one unbroken, seamless
garment for the web of being.

Dwell in this knowledge for a few moments, and then
move your body slightly, open your eyes, and come back
when you feel ready.

Changing Patterns in the Human Energy Field

As you gain experience in working with the human energy
field, you may realize that human energies have a tendency, as do
more material energies, to gather into groups or levels so that patterns result. These patterns relate significantly to functional attributes such as behavioral patterns, emotional dispositions, and
moods.

For instance, the energy field of a person who is depressed may
be perceived by you, the healer, as spiritless, unresponsive, heavy,
and logy in the areas around the heart and solar plexus. The accompanying effect that you yourself feel may be dejection and
discouragement.

Patterns of other illnesses also are energetically distinct. You
may feel pronounced heat in the healee's energy field over inflam-
mations and infections. You may sense specific engorgement or
pressure in the energy field with problems of fluid and electrolyte
imbalance such as in edematous tissue. Curious feelings of coolness
or emptiness may accompany problems of the circulatory system.

There are also patterns of energy-flow rhythmicity, "texture" of the energy field, and other subtle variations of energy that are very difficult to describe clearly. Your perception of these patterns, of course, is commensurate with your own sensitivity and experience as a healer. However, a gross sense of an energy pattern is not difficult for even a beginner to pick up, based on the cues of heat, cold, pressure, and so on.

If you then go on to use the principle of opposites—to "cool" the heat, "release" the pressure, and so on—the symptoms of the infection will lessen, the edema will reduce, and the skin will pinken and flush in response to the increased circulation. It is apparent that Therapeutic Touch does the right thing, because of the return to normalcy; however, it is equally apparent that we really don't know why this happens.

Unruffling the Energy Field

The "texture" of the healee's field may make itself known to the energy centers of your hands in a distinctive way. You may sense the texture, or structural quality, as being rough, agitated, entangled, or disorganized. This unevenness feels as though the energy field's surface is wrinkled or ruffled, whereas ideally the energy flow should be smooth, uniform, and even—in essence, unruffled. "Unruffling," in fact, is the name given to the procedure of smoothing this unevenness by one of my students, and this name has proved to be so appropriate that it continues to be used.

Unruffling clears the energy field so that its texture feels free of the "ruffles" and flows smoothly. Energy patterns can be shifted or moved to the periphery of the healee's energy field where, if they are not too ingrained in the stuff of the energy field itself, they will dissipate.

Ruffled areas are clearly demarcated within the energy field. When you find these ruffled areas during the assessment:

1. Place your hand chakras in the patterned areas in need of unruffling, the palms of your hands turned outward, toward the periphery of the healee's field.

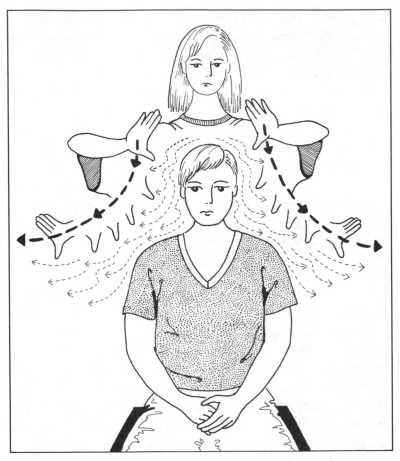

FIGURE 7. Unruffling the Energy Field

2. Now move your hands outward, toward the field periphery. Move both hands as one, with a lateral or somewhat downward sweep of your arms. (See figure 7.)

In some persistent cases, three or four of these sweeps may be necessary to move the ruffled area. The way you know whether more sweeps are needed is by reassessing the area after you have done the unruffling. Reassessment, in fact, should be done after every attempt to rebalance the energy field. If you pick up the same cue, the inference is that you have not adequately rebalanced the healee's energy field.

Unruffling the energy field is very effective in facilitating energy flow. It has a cooling effect, for through its use an elevated temperature can be reduced. It is also useful in clearing decongested areas of sluggish energetic flow such as occur in upper respiratory infections. Unruffling momentarily returns the stuff of the healee's energy field to a more normal state. If you as the healer are sensitive to this moment, memory of its "feel" can act as a model for the energy state of well-being to which you are helping the healee to return. You can then refer to this memory from time to time in your attempt to rebalance the healee's energy field.

As in the other Therapeutic Touch practices, unruffling is done in a general head-to-foot direction. However, there are a few exceptions. For instance, with an extremity that has dependent (pooling) edema, it has proven to be more successful to unruffle in an upward direction in the field overlying the edematous tissue. Start at the end of the extremity—the hand or the foot—and unruffle the overlying energy field upward, toward the head of the healee, rather than downward. There have never been any untoward effects from unruffling. However, since there have been no controlled studies of this practice, as a precaution unruffling should be done no higher than the upper abdomen in cases of edema.

In the past, I have reported on a case of edema in a leg in which Therapeutic Touch reduced the leg circumference by half an inch with only twenty minutes of treatment. In another case of leg edema, Therapeutic Touch reduced the swelling so much that the leg circumference went from 58 centimeters (approximately 23 inches) to 53 centimeters (approximately 21 inches) in twenty-four hours under controlled conditions. There have been other, comparable reports over the years.

The act of unruffling frees bound energy. It also can be used to:

- Facilitate energy flow
- Break up energy patterns, such as congestion

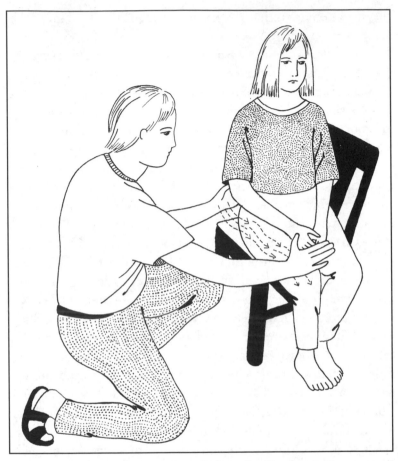

FIGURE 8. Facilitating Movement of

- Reestablish rhythm in the healee's energy field
- Cool, in situations such as elevated temperature
- Move patterned energy within the field
- Knit together the energy field

It is obvious from these seemingly divergent results of unruffling that it is intentionality, rather than the positioning of the hands, that is significant in Therapeutic Touch.

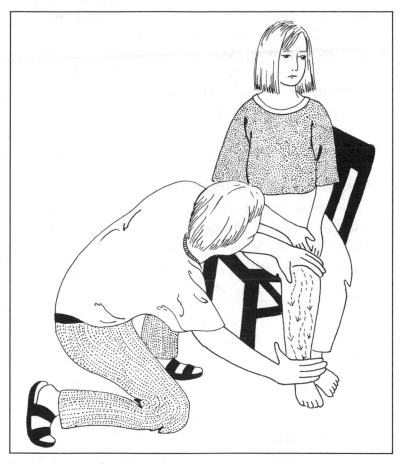

Energy Down the Lower Extremities

Using the Skeleton to Guide Energy Flow

Another technique to move or repattern energy is one I use particularly when there is pain related to skeletal fractures. I got the idea from Ayurvedic medicine, an ancient mode of medical practice that is based on Hindu teachings in the Vedas. This ancient literature suggests that bones act as storage sites for *prana*, a Sanskrit term for the energy that underlies the organization of the life process. I wondered whether this stored prana could be intentionally activated to help reduce congested areas around pain sites. Therefore, I developed a technique to move the congested energy along or through the long bones of the extremities involved in pain. As in everything connected with Therapeutic Touch, it begins with you centering and maintaining a centered state of consciousness. Then:

1. Place one hand on or near the site in the healee's energy field overlying the joint above the pain site. Position the other hand on or near the joint below the pain site.

2. In a manner similar to that used in Experiential Exercise 7, interpenetrate the energy field and direct the flow of prana or life energy from your hand energy center positioned over the upper joint (the joint nearest the trunk of the healee's body) through the pain site and into the lower joint on the extremity.

3. Use the hand chakra, or energy center, positioned at the lower joint as an indicator of whether the intentional energy flow is running to it. In a manner resembling that used in Experiential Exercise 8, "listen" or become sensitive to any increased energetic impingement on this chakra. The major difference between this technique and Experiential Exercise 8 is that in this technique the two hands do somewhat different things: One hand chakra sends or directs the energy flow down the long bone while the other hand chakra senses or receives the intentionally directed energy flow at the site of the lower joint. In the exercise, separate people performed these two different functions.

4. Once your lower hand chakra senses a change or difference in energy flow, and you feel that an increased or more vibrant flow is sustained, shift the hand that was at the upper joint to the site of the second joint. Simultaneously, move your other hand from this second joint to

a third, even lower joint, or to a foot or hand if there are no other joints in the extremity. Again direct the energy flow downward with the chakra of the upper hand and try to sense with the other hand chakra whether the flow is reaching the lower joint.

5. As before, wait until you are aware of an increase or change in the energy flow before you move on. You may find that some light unruffling down the extremity will facilitate the lessening or eradication of pain.

6. If necessary, repeat the procedure. Then, if the healee still experiences no relief, do Therapeutic Touch to an area of the trunk of the body that is toward the spinal column from the uppermost joint of the extremity; then work down the extremity again. However, do not extend the session beyond the recommended twenty to twenty-five minutes. If there is no relief after this time, refer the healee to some other appropriate avenue of therapy.

Figure 8 illustrates the use of this technique in the lower extremities. Refer to figure 9 and the following directions for an example of how to perform this technique in the case of shoulder pain.

1. Place one hand chakra at the shoulder and the other at the elbow. From your energy center at the shoulder, direct prana to the elbow. When the sense of energy flow is received at the elbow, move each hand down one joint.

2. Direct energy from the hand chakra now at the elbow toward the wrist. Meanwhile, sense the energy flow with the hand chakra positioned at the wrist.

Interfacing with Other Modalities

In practice, you may want to modulate the energies as well as direct them. You also will find that Therapeutic Touch neatly interfaces with other therapeutic methods, including those that are

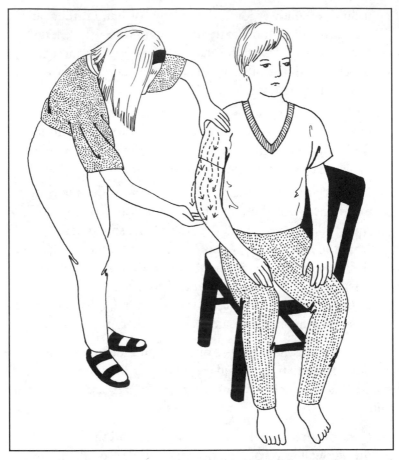

FIGURE 9. Moving Congested

traditional such as shiatsu and acupressure, the more current techniques such as biofeedback and imagery, and many of the formal practices in medicine and nursing. Therapeutic Touch reaches deeply into human dynamics for the ground upon which it works. However, there are limits to what Therapeutic Touch can do, so it is recommended that you recognize these limits and supplement your work with appropriate other modalities, should they be necessary for the healee's well-being.

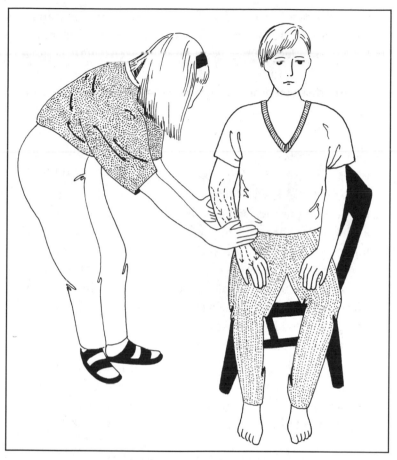

Energy in the Shoulder Area

A Review of Techniques

Following is a review of the directions for Therapeutic Touch techniques discussed so far, with some additional notes:

1. Begin the practice of Therapeutic Touch by making your healee comfortable in a seated or lying position. Stand or sit nearby in a position that is comfortable for you.

2. Take a few moments to quietly center your consciousness, then try to maintain this state of centeredness throughout

the entirety of the session. If you lose this state, maintain your composure; simply step aside or turn away from the healee for a few moments and regain a sense of quietude. Then, if you can, go on with the session. However, if you are too distracted, it is best not to continue. Try again at another time, or refer the healee to someone else who can be of help.

3. After centering, do an assessment of the healee's energy field. Then use whichever of the rebalancing techniques you judge to be appropriate.

4. From time to time, reassess the healee's energy field to evaluate the effect of the energy work. When you no longer pick up cues, it is an indication that the time has come to stop. Under any conditions, do not continue Therapeutic Touch beyond twenty to twenty-five minutes until you have enough experience to spot the signs of energy overload: restlessness, irritability, increasing anxiety, and perhaps hostility or pain.

5. It is very useful to let the healee rest for ten to fifteen minutes after the session. This short period of relaxation helps to ground or stabilize the energies. Frequently the healee will fall asleep, which is regenerative in itself.

Conventions and Cautions

In attempting to rebalance the healee's energy, maintaining rhythm in your movements is essential. What is important in Therapeutic Touch is not so much the amount or intensity of the energy you send to the healee but your ability to integrate the healee's energies into a synchronous flow.

Throughout the session, remain sensitive to cues in the healee's energy field. As noted previously, as you continue this human-energy-field interaction, a natural, deeper engagement between your energy field and that of the healee occurs. In my jargon, you go more *inth*—into a private dimension that is beyond the simple three dimensions of the physical plane. As this occurs, your concomitant increased sensitivity to the healee's energy field frequently gives you an opportunity for a series of rapid reassessments of the field. These reassessments either give you clues about how to continue or, when there are no longer any cues, indicate that it is time to conclude the session.

It bears repeating that an entire session should not take more than twenty to twenty-five minutes. It is actually possible to overdose on energy; therefore, it is important to stay aware of a healee's limits and possible idiosyncrasies. Because a healee's idiosyncrasies are very individualized, you may not be aware of them until you experience them. Therefore, a useful rule is to underdo the therapeutic interaction rather than overdo it. You can always come back at a later time to do another session of Therapeutic Touch.

The progressive signs of energy overload to be aware of include increasing restlessness, irritability, and anxiety that may be expressed as hostility or felt as pain by the healee. The idea that pain can be created with Therapeutic Touch may be surprising. However, you can readily demonstrate the reality of such pain by having someone work on you without regard to your own tolerance. The more sensitive you are, the more quickly you will get the point that Therapeutic Touch is an actual energy interchange.

Burns are very sensitive to energy overload, so Therapeutic Touch must be done very gently at the site of burned tissue. Do the work for very short periods—two to three minutes at a time—and keep your hands moving so that your hand chakras do not focus energy too intensely at the burn site. It is also a very good idea to modulate the energies by visualizing a color in the royal blue range for burns.

To demonstrate on yourself what a concentration of human energy feels like, try the following:

1. Take a moment to center your consciousness.

2. Bring your hands up to the level of your ears and set up an energy field between your hands the same way you did in Experiential Exercise 7.

3. Once you feel the build-up of the energy field, simultaneously move both hands an inch or two to your left. Then, still maintaining the field, move both hands an inch or two to your right.

4. Repeat this back-and-forth maneuver several times at a moderate rate of speed, paying close attention to what is happening to your ear drums.

Can you feel your ear drums respond to the moving field, being pulled first one way and then the other? Imagine what this might feel like to a baby with an ear infection. If you lack the imagination, try this demonstration again on yourself when you have a head cold. The need to be gentle and maintain sensitivity to the healee will quickly become apparent. As noted previously, body fluids and electrolytes seem to be very sensitive to Therapeutic Touch.

As a final word of caution, I suggest that you yourself not be too open in human energy interactions. Do not allow energies that we admittedly do not fully understand to sweep you away. When you consistently practice Therapeutic Touch, you will feel more vital, vigorous, and integrated. Do not use this mood carelessly; ground these energies and let them work for you in a strengthening, positive way.

The best way to ground yourself is to maintain a centered state of consciousness as an entire lifestyle. This way, the energies feed into higher levels of yourself. However, there are also several physical methods of grounding yourself. You can actually sit on the ground in the lap of Mother Earth. Or you can sit or walk on the sands by the sea. Or you can lean up against a tree, particularly a coniferous tree. Nature is very generous in helping us human beings regain a sense of equilibrium.

Lastly, be alert to the psychological effects of such a highly personalized interaction as Therapeutic Touch. Identification, projection, transference, and counter-transference, which may occur in any powerful psychological interaction, are also possibilities in the healer-healee relationship.

Working with a Partner

Because each of us needs a wide range of knowledge to act in a wise and compassionate manner in these complex times, it is useful to work with a partner or colleague in your practice of Therapeutic Touch. Much of what you will learn about the daily practice of Therapeutic Touch is experiential. Therefore, once you understand the underlying principles, you will learn more from your own mindful involvement in this human energy interaction than I could teach you on paper. Because of this, the opportunity to exchange ideas and experiences with another student of Therapeutic Touch practice can be invaluable.

Working with another practitioner on a healee, therefore, can

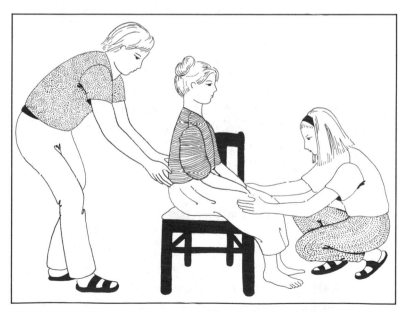

FIGURE 10. Doing Therapeutic Touch with a Partner

be mutually useful for the healers. It is also very important that the interaction be just as useful for the healee. Not only do the healers involved in the therapeutic interaction become sensitive to the healee's energy field, but the healee may also become sensitive to the healers' energy fields. In such a delicate network, therefore, it becomes important for the two healers to closely synchronize their efforts on the healee's behalf.

Following is the procedure for yourself and the other healer (see figure 10):

1. Center yourselves, and in the process make a conscious effort to align your consciousnesses closely with each other.

2. Maintaining this mutually focused state, stand with one of you in front and the other in back of the healee and simultaneously assess the portion of the healee's energy field that is within your reach.

3. When both of you are done, switch places and again assess the area of the healee's field that is within your reach. Each of you has now assessed both "sides" of the healee's energy field.

4. Step aside and quietly discuss your findings between yourselves. Decide upon a plan for rebalancing the healee's energy field. A useful procedure to follow is to designate which of you will direct, modulate, or repattern the energies, and which of you will act as the assistant by moving and grounding the energies (that is, facilitating the flow of energy downward toward the ground) and so on.

In case one of you picked up a cue to which the other healer was not sensitive, the one of you who picked up the cue should do whatever you judge to be appropriate to rebalance the healee's field. The other one of you can assist and support this person's work by conducting the energy being projected through the healee's field, stabilizing the energy over appropriate areas, checking whether the energy is exiting smoothly through the foot chakras (as in Experiential Exercise 8) and so on. Interchange your roles as necessary.

Although no harm will be done if each of you assesses the healee in your own individual style, there is a need for the two of you as healers to maintain the same rhythm of movement as you rebalance the energy field of the healee. As a matter of fact, working rhythmically is a key to success at this stage of the Therapeutic Touch interaction. In practice, since both of you are maintaining a state of centeredness, this close rhythmic coupling will occur naturally, the two of you acting as one, the quiet interweaving of your movements resembling an elegant and stately dance.

Systems Most Sensitive to Therapeutic Touch

It is very helpful to have a clear understanding of the possible physiological effects of Therapeutic Touch. An extensive review of nearly two decades of reports on Therapeutic Touch by health professionals from around the world indicates that the physiological system most sensitive to Therapeutic Touch is the autonomic nervous system (ANS). The ANS is divided into two branches, the parasympathetic and the sympathetic nervous systems. Activation of the sympathetic nervous system results in general excitation. The parasympathetic has a more specific effect on the body; for instance, it acts to relax smooth muscle, decrease heart rate, and increase gastrointestinal functioning. In a continual process of sensitive feedback, each works to limit or control the other's functions. The effect is an "automatic" regulation of the vital activities of daily living, including the visceral, circulatory, and glandular processes. These processes operate in such harmonic synchrony that they function without an individual having to think about them. In contradistinction, the central nervous system activates voluntary functions through the cortex in the upper cap of the brain; it evaluates information about the environment through the subcortical division of the midbrain, basal ganglia, and attached spinal cord.

Disorders related to the parasympathetic branch of the ANS

are focalized, while disorders resulting from hyperactivation of the sympathetic branch occur in many places in the body at the same time. The review indicates that Therapeutic Touch is most useful for psychosomatic illnesses, which are often reflections of autonomic nervous system dysfunction. Today, psychosomatic illness accounts for an estimated 70 percent of the health problems of the world; it is pandemic in these stress-laden times.

The systems next most sensitive to Therapeutic Touch are the lymphatic and circulatory systems. As noted earlier in reference to the rapid effects of Therapeutic Touch on edema, the fluid and electrolyte balances in the body are very responsive to Therapeutic Touch. Also sensitive is the peripheral vascular system. This is evidenced by the characteristic slight flush of the healee's skin, particularly on the face and neck, within the first four minutes of Therapeutic Touch practice. This pinking of the skin, which is frequently generalized over the whole body, occurs without the healer making contact with the healee's body, so it seems indeed to be an energy-field effect.

The system next most affected by Therapeutic Touch is the musculoskeletal system. Particularly responsive in this category are bone fractures. Healees feel a characteristic warmth during Therapeutic Touch that is not on their skin as in kinesthetic (contact) touch, but rather deep within their tissues. This deep warmth is felt even through unwieldy, heavy plaster casts.

There are other systems that are significantly responsive to Therapeutic Touch only with respect to certain disorders. One of these is the collagen system. The various forms of arthritis, for instance, are sensitive to Therapeutic Touch, but other collagen disorders, such as lupus, are not. There is also a limited range of effectiveness of Therapeutic Touch with endocrine disorders. It works very well with thyroid dysfunctions and with problems of the adrenals. It also works well with certain problems of the reproductive system, notably the female reproductive system during pregnancy. However, there have not been significant results with either the pancreas (for example, in diabetes) or the pituitary gland.

There are some strange results with respect to the central nervous system. Paraplegics, even with severances high on the spinal cord, report that they can actually feel the specific areas upon which Therapeutic Touch is being done, even though their skin is not being touched and pressure is not being applied. When Therapeutic Touch is done without skin contact (so that all work is done in the energy field) to wounds that have raw sensory nerves exposed, healees state that they feel pain at the site if the healer's hands are kept there without moving for too long.

The results of Therapeutic Touch with psychological disorders are mixed. Several excellent therapeutic interactions have occurred for persons with manic depression; some occurring during the manic stage have been quite dramatic. There have also been surprisingly good results with catatonic adults and hyperkinetic children. Three catatonic persons, when they returned to consciousness, knew which nurses had been doing Therapeutic Touch with them. This in itself can make one pause to examine life-long assumptions. Such wonder is compounded by similar reports on people who have had cerebral vascular accidents (strokes) and been in deep comas. When they have come out of their comas, they, too, have identified the nurses who treated them with Therapeutic Touch. However, the results of treating people with other psychological problems such as schizophrenia have not been significantly successful thus far.

Finally, Therapeutic Touch has been helpful for only certain aspects of some disorders. For persons with autoimmune deficiency syndrome (AIDS), success has been primarily with the accompanying opportunistic infections and side effects, not with AIDS itself. Elevated temperatures are reduced, and there is some success in clearing pleural effusion and quieting the restlessness that is often part of the clinical picture. At the time of this writing, there is only one well-reported instance of clearing of Kaposi's sarcoma. However, more understanding is coming with time and experience.

There has been limited and mixed success using Therapeutic Touch on persons with Parkinson's syndrome and Alzheimer's disease; however, the one useful result that has occurred in both of these disorders has been the clearing of accompanying agitation.

Several Krieger's Krazies using Therapeutic Touch in hospices throughout the United States and Canada have reported a reduction of pain in people with cancer. They have also consistently reported that when Therapeutic Touch is done in the final stages of cancer, a serene acceptance of the transition of consciousness is apparent in the healee. There has also been success in stabilizing persons in earlier stages of cancer who are undergoing chemotherapy or radiation treatments. I find it most useful to start Therapeutic Touch about a week before the series of treatments is scheduled to begin and then to continue two or three times a week during the series. This stabilizes and supports the healees so that they seem not to experience nausea and vomiting.

It will be apparent to you by now that the techniques of Therapeutic Touch are not difficult to learn. Therefore, upon request, the basic techniques can be taught to relatives and friends of persons who are ill. There are many good reasons for doing this, but high on my list is the unfortunate fact that we, in this time of pride in our objectivity, have a very hard time saying, "I'm sorry" or conveying love for those we hold dear. We hold back with a kind of dull but persistent indifference that defies later rationalization. Sometimes, however, insight prevails when loved ones are ill, and the opportunity to express our deeper feelings can be incorporated into the practice of Therapeutic Touch. Even at a nonverbal level, this act of compassionate concern carries the message.

Besides being a medium for personal expression, Therapeutic Touch is a human potential that can be actualized by virtually everyone willing to undertake the self-discipline called upon for this system of journeying within. This was brought home to me quite powerfully in a letter from one woman stating, "I thought to touch her one last time, to remember her as she was; I didn't know I could heal."

This woman described how she came to do Therapeutic Touch on her dying mother. Day by day she continued the practice, and in a remarkably short time, to everyone's surprise and the daughter's delight, her mother recovered from what had been thought a terminal illness. It is all too obvious that there is still much to be learned about the mysterious complexities of the human condition and the ability to heal. The important lesson for all of us, however, is that we must try.

The Most Reliable Effects of Therapeutic Touch

I have been invited to be a consultant at many hospital grand rounds during which selected patients are visited by teams of hospital staff. During these visits, I have tried to determine which of the effects of Therapeutic Touch are the most reliable. Ranking highest in reliability, in my opinion, is the very rapid relaxation response in the healee. This can be observed two to four minutes after the Therapeutic Touch interaction has begun.

Consistent studies by Herbert Benson and others have shown that the relaxation response facilitates the immune system's defense of the body against foreign agents such as bacteria and viruses. The relaxation response also stimulates the production of brain opiates called endorphins. These are neuropeptides that act to block pain. Because of the relaxation response, children frequently fall asleep, adults often nap, and people of all ages feel refreshed and vitalized during Therapeutic Touch. There is a decrease in tension and a reduction in anxiety. Therefore, it is very helpful to do Therapeutic Touch on persons before procedures about which they feel apprehension, such as during the preinduction of anesthesia in an operating room or dental clinic, or before spinal taps or the administration of intravenous fluids or other infusions. As already mentioned, Therapeutic Touch is supportive during the dying process largely because of the relaxation response that is elicited.

The next most reliable clinical effect of Therapeutic Touch is the amelioration or eradication of pain. It is said that people do not as much fear dying as they fear having frequent or intractable pain or, as Dora Kunz has pointed out to me, having the next pain. Recurrent pain has a frustrating and tiring effect on a person, frequently with consequent physical and emotional immobilization. The relief of pain releases the person's attention from unmitigated concern with self. There is restoration of a healthful self-concept, and the person wants to join the world again.

Although Therapeutic Touch is very good at the reduction of pain, it is wise to keep in mind that pain reduction can be the result of a number of other variables. Suggestion can play an important role in the relief of pain. Right behind this in importance is any special preparation or indoctrination given to a patient before treatment, for strong belief in a treatment's effectiveness can counter even equally strong sensations of pain. A lowered anxiety level is also a known correlate of reduced pain, and of course there are many drugs that produce an analgesic effect.

For Therapeutic Touch's third most reliable clinical effect, I would choose the facilitation of the healing process per se. This can be seen most vividly on repeated x-rays or other less dangerous medical imageries of bone fractures. Several replicated studies have shown that callus formation at the fracture site, which is generally expected to be well formed six weeks after the fracture, is in unexpectedly stable condition two and a half weeks after the fracture when Therapeutic Touch is used. This is one of the reasons that Therapeutic Touch is frequently used in the field by knowledgeable ski patrols, emergency medical technicians, and firemen.

Personal Experiences with Therapeutic Touch Practice

As previously noted, in Therapeutic Touch practice, you as the healer have but one major concern: the human energy field. In this energy field, you are trying to do one or several of the following things:

- Facilitate energy flow.
- Remove or break up congestion or pressure in the energy field.
- Dampen the intensity of the energy flow.

- Free up bound energy or blockages in the energy field.
- Synchronize dysrhythmias in the energy flow.
- Repattern, rebalance, or knit together the energy field so that it can once again function as an integrated whole.

In all of these, you must depend on your personal interpretation of subtle cues about the state or condition of the healee's energy field. How do you know that these subjective impressions have external, objective validity? The answer lies in the fact that you must be your own test object. What you do rests upon your individual judgment, and you cannot evade personal responsibility for your decisions. Note this excerpt from the journal of my student Deirdre in the early days of her Therapeutic Touch practice:

> We paired up and practiced sending energy to one another to try out our skill with Therapeutic Touch. I was really unable to feel anything, and so I questioned the reliability of it all. When my partner said that she felt something in my energy field, I was amazed, and so I decided to play games without her knowing about it. I centered myself and randomly turned my vibes on and off—but, b'gosh! she was right there, correctly interpreting my energy flows, on or off, weak or strong, as I sent them!

It cannot be repeated too often that Therapeutic Touch is not a miracle cure for illnesses, but that it does help the healing process. Its practice is quite low key, so its effectiveness may come as a surprise. This is indicated with candor in the following excerpt from the journal of my student Lu:

> I have been shy about using Therapeutic Touch in my professional practice, but today I used it and it was incredible. I am being oriented for a new job, and the person who was orienting me was called at 4 p.m. to see a patient who was withdrawn and had been lying in bed, mute and with his eyes closed, since lunchtime. The nurses said that he had been crying and then suddenly displayed this behavior. No

one, not even those with whom he had been in the closest rapport, had been able to get him to respond.

We went up to his bedside and the nurse who had been orienting me tried to get a verbal response from the patient, but to no avail. I was moved by the man's inability to communicate, and so I centered myself and then reached out and held his hand, meanwhile directing energy of a calm, compassionate nature through the energy of my hand. Then, using that energy as a kind of probe, I tried to search out where I could be of help.

After a few minutes, he opened his eyes and began talking to me, all the time holding onto my hand as if it were a precious object. He then pulled my hand across his body to the shoulder that was farthest from me, and he told me how much pain he had there and how much relief he now felt.

The person orienting me was dumbfounded. She asked me what I had done, because she realized that something had in fact gone on between the patient and myself. I told her and was not surprised when she said that if she had not seen it, she never would have believed it. Frankly, neither would I!

Can therapeutic effects be the result of suggestion? Of course. Suggestion, persuasion, coercion, and expectation are all known placebos. It is said, however, that the most effective placebo is the sight of a doctor or nurse walking through a patient's hospital room door. It is also said that when a placebo (which supposedly is inert or of no known therapeutic value) does have a therapeutic effect, it is an indication that self-healing is at work—so, hurrah for the placebo!

However, what rationalization can we use if suggestion, persuasion, and so on are out of the question, as in the case of newborn babies? Babies may be thought of as essentially being born with a *tabula rasa*—a blank slate. The following account was reported by a nurse named Joanne who worked in a newborn intensive care unit in a large medical center in New York City:

I work in the NICU at ———— Hospital, New York City. On Monday, we had a full-term baby come to the unit without any signs of respiration. Since the baby wasn't breathing at all, he was immediately intubated. It was then found that there was a pneumothorax [a collection of air or gas in the pleural cavity as a result of a perforation through the chest wall], so a chest tube was put into place.

We tried to stabilize the baby without success. After doing CPR [cardio-pulmonary resuscitation] for more than twenty minutes, the order was given to stop and withdraw all support. The ET [endotracheal] tube, the chest tube, the IVs, everything came out, and everybody got ready to sign off.

I picked up the baby, centered myself, and did Therapeutic Touch on him. Within a short time, to my surprise as well as that of everyone who was in the room, the baby started to breathe. The respirations continued as I worked on him. When he appeared to stabilize, he was put back into the monitor, which recorded that his heart rate was back in the 100s. All support was reinstated.

A similar report was made by a nurse named Dinah who worked in a babies' hospital in Oregon. Her experience with resuscitating two newborn infants who had not breathed until she did Therapeutic Touch on them led to the use of Therapeutic Touch as a routine procedure in her hospital.

Are these instances happenstance? I don't think so. My files overflow with similar reports from persons using Therapeutic Touch in many parts of the world. Its practice does seem to be a very natural human potential. And you do not have to be in the health professions to practice it. There are some legal precautions as well as health safeguards, both of which will be discussed in a later chapter but, generally speaking, anyone can do Therapeutic Touch who has the compassion to help others and the intelligence to practice in a conscious, mindful manner.

Therapeutic Touch has a wide appeal and a broad spectrum of uses. A small sampling of the participants at a recent

Therapeutic Touch workshop indicates this. There was a journalist who had come to do a story on me, but stayed after the interview because he realized there was something in the workshop that he could use to help his disabled son. A person in telecommunications was there who wanted to teach Therapeutic Touch to some people in his office who, like himself, had incipient ulcers. An architect had come because he was studying how people use their bodies sensitively. A horticulturist's objective in taking the workshop was to learn how to do Therapeutic Touch to his plants. There was an actor who had found the human-energy-field techniques of Therapeutic Touch useful for making his projection of emotions to the audience more effective. A high school teacher had been requested by her teenage students to learn Therapeutic Touch and then teach it to them. Two special-education teachers were already teaching it to their students in a nearby state prison program. There also were two senior citizens who had come as representatives from their community of elders; this community wanted to include Therapeutic Touch practices at a hospice where they volunteered their services. And then there was a middle-aged couple who wanted to learn Therapeutic Touch—"just in case."

Over the years, the experiences with Therapeutic Touch of several thousand (more than thirty-seven thousand at this writing) health professionals have demonstrated to me that there are underlying experiential commonalities in its practice.[5] These commonalities suggest that there are natural principles at work in this therapeutic interaction.[6] Therefore, a colleague, Patricia Winstead Fry, and myself conceived of a system to measure levels of Therapeutic Touch practice. We named it the Self-Evaluation of Therapeutic Touch Scale (SETTS).[7] Several of Krieger's Krazies have used SETTS as a model to analyze their journal entries. A SETTS form is contained in appendix 2 for you to use in evaluating your own process as a healer.

A good example of how the healing intentionality underlying Therapeutic Touch can affect one's life is found in the following extracts from Mary Ann's journal:

These successes with Therapeutic Touch have affected me profoundly, and I have found a peacefulness and purposefulness in life through my ability to help those I "touch." After I have centered and am working on the ill person, I feel that I am, in a sense, in a different "place" than my usual physical surroundings. Activity in the environment continues as before, but with little effort I am able to "tune it out." It is as if I am alone with the ill person, and I have a deep knowledge of the task to be performed. The quiet is peaceful, and the serenity seems to touch me physiologically as well as emotionally. I am aware of my hands, but only in the sense of them being extensions that work in concert with my other sensitivities toward the end of meeting the needs of the ill person.

After the assessment, I feel myself getting "stronger" (for want of a better word). I have more confidence and my respirations are quieter, deeper, and slower than usual. I have a sense of inner plenitude that I cannot explain, except to say that I know it to be a feeling within me, not "out there." I do not understand these phenomena, but I know that I experience similar feelings when I sit quietly in church and let that peaceful atmosphere envelop me.

When I feel an "evenness" in the healee's energy field, I conclude the therapy with the certainty that I have been able to help. I am aware of an increase in my own energy level, and a feeling of joyfulness. It is not the giddiness that accompanies anxiety or euphoria, but a quiet joy.

My memory serves me well after doing Therapeutic Touch. I can recall with exceptional clarity the details of the experience. The calm and serenity that I experience is probably important in the memory process. My thoughts are not cluttered with extraneous information; I consciously know what I'm about when I do Therapeutic Touch. Immediately after the therapeutic session, I can recall fine details, which under other circumstances I might not even notice.

My sense of time is slowed during the act of Therapeutic

Touch. I might spend fifteen or twenty minutes with a person and yet not be aware of the passing of those many minutes at all. This aspect of Therapeutic Touch I find rather extraordinary, because I am usually acutely aware of time and what I can accomplish during its passing.

Recently, when I do Therapeutic Touch, I realize that I am not primarily aware of myself as an individual, but rather as a process. I frequently think of the dream I had in which I experienced a visual imaging of energy in its many forms. During the time when this image comes into focus, I feel that my sensitivity to the energy depletions of the ill person is more acute. I think of the strength and wholesomeness of my own energy complex, and I am at ease somatically, yet purposeful in my "work."

I feel bonded for the period that I am with the ill person. Oddly, though, I do not feel obligated to prolong a session if I wish to leave. This differs significantly from other experiences in which I felt a particular closeness to the patients but had difficulty leaving their presence. Previous to learning about Therapeutic Touch, I usually felt depleted of energy after a close encounter with a patient. Now I feel no loss of energy; I would even say that I feel more energetic!!

Mary Ann's account speaks for itself. However, what about the healee? What is happening within the person who is the recipient of Therapeutic Touch? Judy's sensitive account of her pregnancy and the birth of her little girl lends insight:

During pregnancy and childbirth, I learned a lot about the importance of Therapeutic Touch and of touch in general to the recipient. Specifically, I was healed within two weeks by Dr. Krieger for an anemia that had threatened to prevent me from having a home birth. Although I had read reports of Dr. Krieger's studies on the effect of Therapeutic Touch on hemoglobin (which is deficient in anemia), I had not realized the far-reaching significance that this phenomenon of healing could have for the healee until I experienced it myself.

The anemia was severe and utterly unamenable to my adjustments in diet, supplementation with iron therapy, and other conventional methods. So the doctor refused to sanc tion a home delivery unless there was a dramatic change in my blood picture. I felt that a home birth would be very important to the health and comfort of my baby and myself, and that it would provide an important bonding experience that would affect our relationship for years to come.

That I was able to have this experience, because my hemoglobin responded so significantly to Dr. Krieger's use of Therapeutic Touch for the anemia, filled me with a sense of gratitude and a reverential feeling difficult to describe. It was as if I felt myself to be more closely in touch with the universal life force through this experience. I also had a more optimistic view about life, my place in it, and my ability to overcome obstacles.

The Therapeutic Touch interaction itself seemed to give me a sense of confidence. This confidence was associated with the feeling that someone, in this case Dr. Krieger, cared enough about my well-being to help me in this manner. This act of healing on Dr. Krieger's part gave me support at a time when I needed it badly. During the pregnancy I had experienced many doubts about my abilities to be a good mother. I had been afraid that I might be awkward or insensitive or that I would not experience the essential mother-child bond. However, when the child was presented to me at the moment of birth, I felt the most intense feelings of love and warmth that I had ever known.

In the following days, as I held and cared for my baby, I felt an unanticipated confidence and security. I feel that this sense of confidence may be strongly related to the Therapeutic Touch interaction, the loving care that I had received during labor, and the exquisite bonding experience afforded by the home birth.

A less intense, but just as specific description of the human-energy interchange is conveyed in Laura's log:

Michelle worked on me last week. I was in a very low energy state and had a severe tension headache; also I wanted to experience Therapeutic Touch.

After centering, she began with an assessment, during which time she found a decrease in energy over my right shoulder (which is where my headache felt as though it was coming from) and also a break in energy flow in the area around my head. I didn't feel any of this, but when Michelle began to work in these areas, I did feel a decided energetic shift.

She then worked on balancing the energy between my left and right sides and, in general, getting the energy to flow smoothly and synchronously. There was one moment when she was directing energy to my back that I distinctly felt something "jump" in there, and when I mentioned this to Michelle she said that she had felt it too. My sense of it was that she had gotten "through" at that moment.

From then on I could feel her hands more clearly and the heat that they generated (although they weren't making contact with my skin). When she finished, my headache was gone and I felt more fluid and balanced. Even the sense of "weight" on my shoulders (the favorite home of my anxieties!) felt much lighter.

The sense of heat that Laura described is a specific perceived characteristic of healing, as was previously noted. It is not the heat one feels when a hot stove is touched or a finger is passed through a flame; that is, it is not felt with the skin but within the deep tissues. Two excerpts from clinical notes graphically describe this sense of heat:

With my eyes closed, I lay flat on the bed. Even without looking at the nurse who was doing Therapeutic Touch, I felt two waves of heat coming toward me. The sense of heat was not unpleasant or uncomfortable, and it seemed to be located within my body. Her hands did not touch my body, but as they moved I could feel the sensation of heat keep pace with the direction that her hands moved. In surprise, I

opened my eyes and watched the tracking of her hand placement to the heat that I felt deep in my tissues.

When she then proceeded to place one hand under my
right side and the other hand opposite it, above my body,
I could distinctly feel the heat come from the underlying
hand and travel through my body toward the overlying hand.
At first my whole body reacted, like a mild shock, but then
I felt myself gently relaxing until I almost fell asleep.

As the nurse continued Therapeutic Touch, the pain
became less and less. When she finished, the pain all through
my body, but particularly in my ribs, was almost gone. I lay
there quietly, relaxed and at the edge of sleep, for a period
of one hour—the first time since the operation—the
penetrating heat remaining within my tissues during that
time.

Linda's description indicates the commonality of this perception of heat or movement during Therapeutic Touch:

On December 8, Dr. Krieger placed the palms of her
hands several inches above the area of my adrenal glands,
and I felt a distinct force flowing from her hands to me; I
actually felt energy from the area of her hands penetrating
my body. What I felt was neither heat nor pressure; I would
describe what I felt as the gentle bursting of little effervescent bubbles. . . . It was a distinct and readily identifiable
form of energy, and I really wasn't expecting it to be so.

What are the limits of Therapeutic Touch? Not knowing as
yet the full extent of intervening or imperceptible variables, it is
hard to judge just where to focus observations and analysis.
However, the most obvious places would be the two major transition phases of the life process, birth and death.

My thoughts first went in this direction during a study I did
on Therapeutic Touch in 1982. In this study, I taught husbands
how to do Therapeutic Touch on their pregnant wives during the
third trimester of pregnancy, between the seventh and ninth
months. This study had a most unexpected finding: During the

husbands' assessments of their wives' energy fields, the husbands could distinguish with their hand chakras between the energy fields of the growing fetuses and those of the mothers.

After the reliability of this startling finding was assured, I began to realize that a baby does not spring forth from the womb fully formed, like Venus arising from the froth of the sea. Apparently, before birth, a great deal occurs in the baby's energy field as well as in the baby's physical development. What the father feels when assessing his pregnant wife is the singular energy dynamic of the fetus, a living entity in itself.

Death, the other end of the life spectrum, is equally mysterious to us. When Therapeutic Touch is given to persons who are dying, the transition into death is remarkably peaceful. In the words of Judith, a nurse who did Therapeutic Touch to a five-year-old boy dying of leukemia, "Even death was beautiful." When Cathy and Betsy, a nurse and an occupational therapist, did Therapeutic Touch to their friend, an elderly Benedictine monk who was dying of cancer, the brothers at the priory were so impressed by the calm acceptance and tranquility that seemed to attend this interaction that they asked Betsy and Cathy to teach them Therapeutic Touch, which, of course, they did.

Putting It Together

Therapeutic Touch is a very rich experience, both for the healer and the healee. Following is a review of the major processes and concepts of Therapeutic Touch discussed so far.

Centering

The act of centering is the point of entry for the healing process, and this state of consciousness is maintained throughout the therapeutic engagement. It is a state of deep, inner quietude, a state in which, although you are in time, you are not bound to time or restricted by it. In centering, you touch on a sense of time that flows effortlessly and evenly, rather than with the staccato spurts of attention usual in these stress-laden times. Dora Kunz has said that centering "brings energies to a focal point in the heart and a sense of peace throughout ourselves."

Centering acts as an arena for self-discovery and a bridge to the transpersonal. Through it you can be in touch with the matrix of your potentialities. It allows you to be fully present for those who are weak, in pain, or enmeshed in fear. However, the personal experience of centering also allows you to know with resolute certainty that these sorrowful conditions are finite, transitional, and of limited conscious awareness. It permits the acknowledgment that yes, you are whatever may be the circumscribed conditions of your life, but also that you are much more. It is in such a context that order and meaning for your life are found and appreciated.

Assessment

The assessment phase of Therapeutic Touch provides the clues to the healee's problems. The cues you pick up in the energy field of the healee are subjective and therefore may or may not be the same as the cues perceived by another person assessing the same energy field. From the Eastern frame of reference, cues such as heat, cold, pressure, and so on may relate to any one or a combination of five different subsystems of life energy thought to affect everything from the body's nutrition to its neurological system to emotions of panic, altruistic love, and so on. From this perspective, it seems reasonable to assume that there are many individual sensitivities to human energy. No one person's perception is more right than another's. What is important is that we each be willing to test our sensitivities to create a reality base upon which to help or heal.

Energy Rebalancing

The healthy rebalancing of an ill person's energy is the goal of Therapeutic Touch. The brunt of the therapeutic effort is twofold: to be a human energy support system, and to consciously use that support toward facilitating the healee's energy flow and stimulating his or her immunological system. Based on these goals, in the end it is the healee who in fact heals his or her own self.

Energy Modulation

In modulating human energy, you are primarily working with the healee's energy field. Your attention is on one of the following: dampening, toning down, or sedating the energy flow; vitalizing, quickening, strengthening, or stimulating the energy flow; or establishing rhythm, synchronous blending, or harmonic patterning of the multilevel streaming of the energy.

Energy Unruffling

When unruffling the energy field during Therapeutic Touch, you are smoothing, clearing, or freeing the energy from disturbances that cause turbulence in the field. Such upsets are frequently of a psychodynamic nature. They are due to such things as emotional stress, ambivalence of impulse, anxiety, or fear. If unattended, these energy symptoms frequently cross over into psychosomatic dysfunctions such as hypertension. Unruffling the energy field facilitates a change that is requisite for health. It can also involve an explicit transfer of energy from stress points such as the muscles at the back of the neck. Energy overload can be moved down the long bones of the extremities or down the spine to the periphery of the healee's energy field, where it can dissipate.

In addition to Therapeutic Touch, the healee may require health reeducation or counseling. If you are not qualified in these areas, do not hesitate to refer the healee to a reliable therapist, for is is as important to recognize underlying emotional aspects of an illness as it is to get rid of physical symptoms.

It is most important to put the principles outlined in this chapter into practice. More information without experience will not necessarily make you a better practitioner of Therapeutic Touch. As noted previously, the understanding and judicious use of Therapeutic Touch rests on a base of individually experienced knowledge gained through its practice on living beings. Without playing it through yourself, you will have only the words but none of the music.

To help you with your practice, I am including in Experiential Exercise 10 a Therapeutic Touch Post-Assessment Data Sheet, which is a suggested outline of information for you to gather as you do Therapeutic Touch to a healee. The format of this outline assumes that, at least in the early stages of your practice, you are working with one or more other practitioners. As previously noted, sharing information and experiences with others is one way to significantly expand your range of experiential knowledge about Therapeutic Touch practices. However, the form can easily be revised should you decide to work alone.

In addition to this information form, there is also a companion form in the exercise, the Therapeutic Touch Healee Evaluation Form, which is to be filled in by the healee. Both of these forms are meant to be filled in at the end of a session. Their purpose is to give your team a source of objective feedback from which each participant can learn.

EXPERIENTIAL EXERCISE 10

Post-Assessment Data Sheet and Healee Evaluation Form

Post-Assessment Data Sheet (to be used by the team of healers)

Name of Healee _____ Date _____

After your team has assessed the healee, make sure that he or she is in a comfortable and safe position, then withdraw out of hearing range and discuss your experiences among yourselves. Come to a group decision about the following questions:

1. How did the healee describe his or her problem?

2. Where on the healee's body are the physical location(s) of the problem? Does the healee's posture give any hint about the state of his or her health? Are there any scars or marks on the healee's body?

3. Are there any significant emotional components of the problem? How do they present themselves?

4. Are there any idiosyncrasies or unique factors about the healee that might be of significance to his or her problems?

5. Are there any irregular or unexpected findings?

6. What cues were picked up? Where in the healee's energy field did they seem to be?

7. In the group's opinion, what is the severity of the problem? Check one:
Acute ———— Chronic ———— Mild ————

8. What is your immediate plan for rebalancing the healee's energy field?

Based upon the group's decision, proceed to do Therapeutic Touch to the healee. At the conclusion, complete the following questions:

1. Did you complete the original plan of treatment, or did something come up during the course of treatment to cause you to deviate from the original plan? What happened?

2. In general, do you think Therapeutic Touch was effective for this healee?

3. Do you think that further Therapeutic Touch sessions are warranted for this healee? If so, what would you do at the next session? What would be your long-term objectives for continued sessions?

4. Would you suggest referrals for this healee? Why?

5. What did you tell the healee at the conclusion of the session?

Healee Evaluation Form (to be filled out by the healee)

After you have rested following your Therapeutic Touch session, please briefly answer the following questions:

1. How do you feel at this time?

2. Do you think the persons doing Therapeutic Touch were helpful to you? In what ways?

3. Do you have suggestions on how they could have been more effective?

   Thank you very much.

———————————————————————————————

Chapter 4

AN ANALYSIS OF THE THERAPEUTIC TOUCH PROCESS

Not knowing what to expect, the young man quieted his wandering thoughts as he had been taught and then reached his hands tentatively toward the periphery of his pregnant wife's body. Without touching her skin, he explored the space three to four inches from her body's surface. A few minutes ago, as he had listened to the instructor describe this assessment phase of Therapeutic Touch, it had seemed to be just part of a silly exercise. He knew his wife better than anyone in the world, and although the touch of her skin drew forth emotional responses of a depth he hadn't realized before their marriage, he was sure that the experience ended when there was no longer contact between them except, perhaps, in the memory of that touch. He now cautioned himself to remain nonjudgmental and to maintain the necessary focused state of consciousness while his hands acted as sensitive antennae to pick up any sense of imbalance in his wife's energy field.

For a few moments, he felt a foreboding sense of the failure he was sure awaited him. But as he was about to withdraw his hands, he felt something that piqued his interest. His attention sharpened, and he became acutely aware of a fine and subtle energy flow between himself and his wife that he had never experienced before. Intrigued, he systematically explored his wife's energy field, not quite understanding what he was feeling but aware of a new level of intimacy and sense of oneness between them.

Now, seemingly of their own accord, his hands continued their searching sweeps through his wife's energy field, picking up previously unnoticed clues about her presence. As he became more accustomed to these fine nuances of her energy flows and rhythms, he thought they seemed familiar, as if he had always known them.

This reverie was abruptly interrupted by a realization that there was a delicate shift in the energy flows his hands were experiencing. The effect of this sudden deviation was more felt than understood. He was aware of a strong contraction in the region of his own heart and simultaneously, it seemed, an upheaval within himself about which he later said, "It just felt like my solar plexus flipped over!" The total experience, however, was suffused with a sense of exhilaration.

As he looked down at his hands, he realized that they were poised over the fundus of his wife's swelling abdomen, and he heard himself saying, "That's my child. I feel my child!" Hearing the rising timbre of his voice, he felt foolish, but a glance at his wife gave him the courage to return his attention to his systematic explorations. For a full minute, he kept his attention focused on the phenomenon he was sensing. Then he raised his eyes to meet his wife's gaze again and said, "Yes, it is the child. It feels different from your energy flow, although it is a part of it, as it is a part of mine."

This story is not science fiction. It is representative of scenes that have occurred with predictive frequency since 1984, when I did a study of husbands performing Therapeutic Touch on their pregnant wives during the third trimester of pregnancy (alluded to in the last chapter).[1] This study has been replicated by professional nurses and registered midwives in both the United States and in Canada. Now this use of Therapeutic Touch is considered routine procedure in many parts of North America.[2]

As I mentioned previously, Dora Kunz and I first developed Therapeutic Touch for persons in the health-care field. However, since these study findings were reported, Therapeutic Touch has been used increasingly by members of the public in the home, workplace, and recreational areas, and I value these questors as a new generation of "Krieger's Krazies."

On the pages that follow, a few of these members of the public share their experiences with Therapeutic Touch. The first is a woman named Annette, the mother of a young child. Cuddled up on a couch in the living room of her house, she writes:

> *Monday, 11 p.m.:* Today I tried Therapeutic Touch out of desperation. Adam, the almost three-year-old who has been trying to put me in a grave since his birth, had another well-timed asthma attack. The slightest cold sets it off. On a night when we stayed out until 3 a.m., he started loud and clear at 4 a.m.
>
> In the morning, after a trip to the pediatrician and one shot, we settled down, expectant of the usual two to four days of wheezing. He's supposed to take somophylline every six hours to keep it under control. But Adam is one of those charmers who refuses to eat anything but beef, potatoes, corn soup, and Cheerios with raisins in them. This morning he refused to drink anything if the medicine had been mixed in it. I even gave him back his bottle, I was that desperate—he dumped it down the sink twice and demanded plain juice.
>
> Between 12 p.m. and 2 p.m., Adam purposely vomited three different doses of medicine, taken under the threat of a return trip to the doctor. He was starting to wheeze quite badly again, so I figured, what the hell, nothing else was working, I might as well give Therapeutic Touch a try.
>
> After convincing him to sit still on the couch (which was fairly easy because he was already lying there crying, "I'm sick, I'm sick!"), I centered as best as I could under the circumstances and tried to assess his energy field. I began at his head and worked toward his chest, trying to clear away the heat I felt at his forehead and lower chest. After a while he started smiling and just lay there quietly. After about ten minutes I felt finished and stopped. Adam relaxed on the couch and drank "just a plain juice bottle." He was a new person.
>
> My mother was visiting and was totally amazed (although she hasn't credited Therapeutic Touch with the

change). This sick, pathetic, whimpering kid was turned into a ball of fire. Adam complained of hunger and ate three bowls of soup (the first food he'd had since Saturday night) and talked nonstop until 9 p.m. He dragged all his cars out and played with them on the floor of the den. He must have had a dozen glasses and bottles of juice and tea. The wheezing was completely gone after another Therapeutic Touch session, and just signs of a light cold remained. He was a totally different child—laughing and playing and into mischief. He must have used up an entire box of tissues as everything loosened up.

Later, my husband came home with a headache, a major catastrophe for him. Steve has a low pain tolerance—the result of being an only child, he says. He announced that he was catching Adam's cold. After hearing how well Adam was, he wanted me to "try your thing" on him.

I did Therapeutic Touch about an hour ago on Steve. He fell asleep! But I felt more heat on the right side of his forehead than on his left, so I woke him up to check. He couldn't remember, but he claimed to feel much better. I'm not sure what happened. There is a good chance that he just felt tired and neglected (my mother and his father are staying with us this week, so it is like Grand Central Station around here). He might have felt better lying down and dozing for half an hour.

Steve is still asleep. I'm not sure if he is doing it to bug me, humor me, or get into the act because he now really believes Therapeutic Touch will help him. . . . At least he didn't take any Tylenol tonight. That is very unlike him; if something is wrong he has got to take a pill. He gave himself an ulcer two years ago by taking aspirins every four hours around the clock for a month during a sinusitis attack. . . . The slightest problem is a calamity to him. He once wrote his last will when he had a virus. . . .

I just went in to check on him and he is sound asleep. I noticed that when I did Therapeutic Touch while he slept, if my hands went near his throat, he swallowed. I tried it quite a few times, making sure that I was not physically touching him—he swallowed every time. Right now he's deeply asleep, and I am tempted to wake him to see how he feels. But if he wakes up and still feels lousy, I'll be spending the next half hour setting up the vaporizer, and so on and so on—and I just don't have the courage!

In a small apartment house, a second woman, Susan, writes in her journal about a neighbor who came home from work with a throbbing tension headache and sought her out for help:

I began my assessment carefully, systematically, running my hands above her head and then toward her feet. It is obvious that she has a slight temperature elevation, but the intensity of "heat" that I feel is even greater along her back and in the region of her shoulder blades. I redirect my energy toward these areas in particular. Within a short while I can tell that she is relaxed: her face is slightly flushed, she is breathing evenly, and her hands are resting quietly in her lap. This is a precious moment—we are one, healer and healee. As I finish the Therapeutic Touch, even before receiving verbal confirmation, I know that I have helped my friend. She reports that the headache and nausea "have just evaporated" and that she now feels a sense of well-being. Although I try to maintain my objectivity, I am elated!

In retrospect, I realize now that my skepticism and rationalizations were all defenses to cover my ignorance. I now know for a fact that Therapeutic Touch can be done, even by me.

Yes, Therapeutic Touch can be done by everyone, even by you. There is a wide range of expertise levels with the practice of Therapeutic Touch, but the key to a high level of expertise is knowledgeable practice motivated by a compassionate concern for the well-being of another. As previously mentioned, it is sometimes also useful for Therapeutic Touch to be used in conjunction with other selected modalities as an extension of professional skills. Anne, an unusual medical social worker from

Canada, writes about a woman who was admitted to the hospital with third-degree burns on both hands:

> I didn't start to do Therapeutic Touch until the day they discovered that the grafts had not taken. On that day, I did two sessions of Therapeutic Touch to her hands and then taught her some visualization and relaxation exercises as "homework" for her to do. The very next morning, the doctor asked me what had happened. He had just examined the patient's hands and noticed that they had started to seed, or heal themselves. Her progress since then has been truly phenomenal. I have done Therapeutic Touch with her daily, and she has now gone home and is able to use her hands again. She comes back on a regular outpatient program for physiotherapy and Therapeutic Touch.

These vignettes portray a variety of Therapeutic Touch practices. There are many hundreds more examples that have been written up and validated that could be included here. However, I am not trying to convince you of the efficacy of Therapeutic Touch— my hope is that you have already been convinced if you have read this far.

The important theme in this small collection of personal notes is that the practitioner was willing to try, even when other therapeutics had failed. These accounts all indicate that the try was worth it. After almost two decades of developing Therapeutic Touch, I will say that Therapeutic Touch, done in the manner that my colleague Dora Kunz and I suggest, is a very useful helping/healing modality and one that is safe for both healer and healee. So I urge you to try it when the need arises.

The importance of trying was brought home to me recently by a note in one of my students' objectives for a course:

> My mother is dying of cancer, and there is so little I can do. But I want to try to help in some way, if only in making her transition a bit easier. Through Therapeutic Touch, I think I will have that opportunity, and I would like to try.

This selection of personal notes involves Therapeutic Touch being practiced by a diverse group of people: a distraught mother, a concerned neighbor, a compassionate health practitioner, and a loving daughter with the courage to try. On the surface, these people have little in common except a need to help, a sense of deep caring, and a compassionate concern for the well-being of another person. However, at a more profound level, each was willing to use herself to knowledgeably intervene as a human support system. This assumes at least two things: each had been willing to learn the techniques of Therapeutic Touch, which requires a measure of self-discipline, and each was willing to consciously—with full awareness—use her own energies in a helping/healing act.

So far, I have dealt primarily with the techniques of Therapeutic Touch. These techniques, as previously noted, do not stand by themselves but reach deeply into the psyche of the practitioner. It is through the conscious use of the psyche, the power of mindful intentionality, and the healing interaction between human energy fields that the vigor and effectiveness of Therapeutic Touch arise.

A Systems Model for the Therapeutic Touch Assessment

What is the nature of the human energy field? My own ability to tackle this query requires analogical thinking, rather than direct perception. Consequently, I find the relativistic quantum theory of new physics useful to gain insight into the nature of energy. Quantum theory holds that all reality consists of energy fields—that 99.9999 percent of the universe is space rather than what we know as solid matter. Quantum theorists say that where energy fields cross, there is evidence of the momentary creation of particles, or matter. Other than these sets of energy fields, "there isn't anything else," says Pagels, a noted authority on quantum theory.[3]

I perceive the human energy field as a large system of incessantly interacting fields, many (perhaps most) of which we are not consciously aware. For instance, at this moment you are a test object for at least two important energy fields: the electromagnetic field, via whose photons you are seeing this page, and the gravitational field, by virtue of which you are probably sitting on a seat rather than levitating to the ceiling. These many energy fields are crucial to the human life process. Where they cross—at the nexus of that intersection—is the human being, the "particle" of living consciousness. In this model, it seems apparent that the human being is sensitive to more energy fields than any other living creature, which is why humans are at the top of the evolutionary ladder. To take the model one step further, it is these constantly shifting, interacting and interrelating energy fields that are the basis of reality.

In Therapeutic Touch, it is to the incessant flow of the healee's energy fields that you as the practitioner look when you are assessing the reality of the healee's condition. This reality is interpreted through indicators such as temperature differentials, pressure gradients, pulsations, "tingles," feelings similar to slight electric shocks, and so on. These indicators occur during the assessment and reassessment phases of Therapeutic Touch.

But how is it that you can pick up such information from the energy field? This is an interesting, exciting, but almost impossible question to answer because we understand so little about the dynamic foundations of the human condition. However, a theoretical model could be created to portray some of the variables involved in this dynamic. Systems theory lends itself most readily to such an analysis. Within such a systems model, the subsystems involved in the Therapeutic Touch assessment process can be specified and a flow sheet can be constructed of the apparent interactions taking place.

Such a flow sheet of human energy subsystems in the Therapeutic Touch assessment is depicted here. With the background of this energy flow being a centered state of consciousness, the flow sheet is interpreted as follows:

Your initial evaluation of the healee arises out of many facets of your memory, which is primarily based in your previous ex-

Flow Sheet of Human Energy Subsystems Used in Therapeutic Touch*

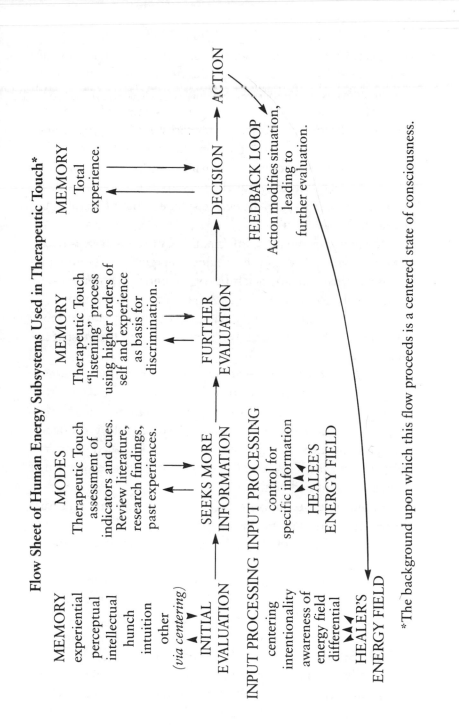

MEMORY
experiential
perceptual
intellectual
hunch
intuition
other
(via centering)
INITIAL EVALUATION →

MODES
Therapeutic Touch assessment of indicators and cues.
Review literature, research findings, past experiences.

SEEKS MORE INFORMATION →

MEMORY
Therapeutic Touch "listening" process using higher orders of self and experience as basis for discrimination.

FURTHER EVALUATION →

MEMORY
Total experience.

DECISION → ACTION

FEEDBACK LOOP
Action modifies situation, leading to further evaluation.

INPUT PROCESSING
centering
intentionality
awareness of energy field differential
HEALER'S ENERGY FIELD

INPUT PROCESSING
control for specific information
HEALEE'S ENERGY FIELD

*The background upon which this flow proceeds is a centered state of consciousness.

periences. Closely coupled with your memory are cues that are perceptual and intellectual. Perceptual cues are those you perceive with your senses, as when you see a person on crutches, or with your imagination, as when you talk by telephone about or to a healee. Intellectual cues arise from processes within your mind, as, for instance, when you infer from the crutches that the healee has a problem with locomotion. You may also have a simultaneous hunch or true intuition about the person's condition. Any or all of these factors give you as the healer a tentative basis for evaluating the healee's condition.

You then seek out more information by becoming sensitive to the indicators and cues in the healee's energy field. As information is gathered, you go back into your memory to accommodate these bits of information. You associate them with what you have previously read about similar energy patterns, or you consider known research findings that might coincide with the present circumstances.

To focus in on the nature of the problem from a human energy perspective, you attentively "listen" with your hands and other energy centers, and you fine-tune your sensitivities to any further clues that may be sensed from the healee's energy field. Once again, you relate any new information to previous knowledge and experience, and you integrate all the data within the perspective of yourself as a unified being.

At this time, you make a decision about how you will treat the healee's condition. However, this is not the end of the assessment process, for as you get more *inth*, that is, as your own energy field interacts sensitively and therapeutically with that of the healee, you will frequently get a more explicit and profound understanding of the dynamic state of the healee's energy field. As necessary, you will then reassess how you can help the healee.

This model is straightforward and, of course, quite linear in its logic. However, it does what it purports to do, which is to graphically outline the significant subsystems involved in the Therapeutic Touch assessment process. It does not delineate the treatment for the healee nor how healing might occur. Such issues demand a more heuristic approach than is now available with our present Western thinking, and of necessity they will have to be put aside at this time. However, you can take comfort in the thought that just as you do not need to know how a car works in order to drive it, so can you use Therapeutic Touch without knowing exactly how its healing processes operate, and, when it is appropriate, it will work in the interest of the healee.

Allies in the Healing Process

The assuredness of Therapeutic Touch's healing effects arises from the fact that within the human body there are many natural allies. There are many levels of energy related to the healing process that can be called upon and reinforced, for, as has been noted frequently, in the end it is the healee who heals himself or herself. These abilities are the recuperative powers of the body, and there are several that can be pinpointed. Prime among them is the immunological system, which is a major apparatus for rebalancing human energies and maintaining their natural harmonics. Helping with this task is the autonomic nervous system, which offers instantaneous, protective, biological reactions to trauma, and the endocrine system, which helps fire off many of these protective reactions and assists with the body's healing process, particularly during a relaxation response.

Recuperation is also a function of the endorphins, enkaphalins, and other neuropeptides throughout the body, which bring pain and its sequelae under the control of the healee. The thalamus, resting in the middle of the brain, also assists by filtering out excessive pain sensations before they come to conscious awareness. One measure of the body's efficiency for healing is the skin, a system in itself that exhibits extremely rapid regeneration. Also quickly regenerative are bone tissue, the liver, and the peripheral nerves.

Therapeutic Touch as a healing process apparently reaches and heightens the effects of all these natural allies. How this therapeutic human-energy interchange occurs is not well understood within the Western, high-tech frame of reference, as was noted above. However, Eastern thought, which is based on inner, experiential knowledge, provides a more humanistic basis for insight into the functioning of human energies and how Therapeutic Touch assists in the healing process.

The Concept of Human Energy

Our knowledge of nature has changed many times over the millennia as sophisticated human understanding has slowly developed out of the seeds of mere curiosity. However, the awesome ability of the body to heal itself—and the awe-inspiring, humane, intentional redirection of healing energies from one individual to another—have riveted attention in all cultures throughout history. The healing energy that is the birthright of all physical organisms (for there is no living thing that cannot heal itself within limitations) has been noted throughout recorded time—in the most ancient of cave paintings, conceived fifteen thousand years ago, and in the computerized retrieval systems of modern hospitals.

The concepts of essential life energy go by a variety of names in different parts of the world, but there are strong correlations among them. From my studies of healing systems, it appears that there are three major perspectives on vital energies that have significantly influenced Western thought: the East Indian, the Chinese, and the Egyptian. In India, the Sanskrit term for vital energy is *prana*. Prana is said to flow through the energy field of the physical body in nonphysical channels called *nadis*. In Pinyin Chinese, this energy, which is described as flowing through a nonphysical network of meridians, is called *qi* or *ch'i*. The ancient Egyptian name for the energetic equivalent of the physical body is the *ka*. This term is still in use, as are the other two.

These traditional views of vital energy have striking commonalities; they are fundamentally consistent with each other. In each culture, knowledge about human energetics is included in the most venerated of ancient writings, so that a case can be supported for a common source of all three major interpretations of vital energy. Underlying this source is an evolving understanding of the human condition itself.

The individual's confrontation with universal forces is more personal within the Indian model. Indian philosophy underscores the deeply embedded karmic (specific cause-effect) relationships of the individual, the disease or limiting condition, and its cure. Foundational to the whole body of Indian thought is a clear declaration of the unitive relationship of all people. Because this idea is consonant with the conceptual basis of Therapeutic Touch, it is useful to study the Indian perspective of human energy systems.

The Indian concept of human energies is succinctly organized in literature extending back to the Rig-Veda of about 2000 B.C. According to this body of experiential knowledge, there are three types of energies concerned with health. These are *prana*, previously mentioned as the vital energy that underlies the organization of the life process; *kundalini*, which is concerned with creative energies in the sense approximated by the psychological term *libido*; and an energy that is somewhat akin to the Greek concept of eros, or love. The Therapeutic Touch process is primarily concerned with prana, although all three subsets of human energy are closely integrated.

In health, prana is in an energy-rich state. As prana flows through its circuitry, the nadis, it acts as a conveyor for *citta*, the psyche's willful, emotional, and intellective functions. In this model, it is citta that puts us in contact with the environment through sensory input. The aim of hatha yoga is the conscious control of citta, so that it flares up as a fire (*hatha* means the violent arrest of the inconsistency and uncertainty of citta). When citta is controlled, illumination or expansion of consciousness is released through one of the major nadis, the *sushumna*. Then the citta gradually becomes purified, leading to serenity (*samadhi*). *Sakti*, an active force, governs this process.

The pranic currents move and circulate through the nadis in a manner related to the sun, the moon, and the condition of the person. The *sushumna*, the principal nadi, is described as running up the lumen or hollow core at the center of the spinal cord "like a thread through the eye of a needle." It is this lumen that in the West is thought to be the remnant of the hollow tube from which both the spinal cord and the brain develop embryonically.[4] In Indian literature, the sushumna is described very precisely as beginning five centimeters above the anus and five centimeters behind the penis in the male, or its embryological equivalent in the female. It then moves to the muladhara chakra at the base of the spine. In Western terms, chakras can be thought of as transformers. They transform various universal energies into energies that are usable by the human being for the functioning of its body. Like the hand chakras mentioned earlier, chakras are situated in what science would call the biofield of the body.

Two other major nadis that function in conjunction with the sushumna are the *ida* and the *pingala*. They start in the same place as the sushumna, but when energized they encircle the spinal-cord energy field in a serpentine fashion. They ascend in opposite directions, each pacing the other. The ida twines to the left; it is pale, lunar, and feminine. The pingala twists to the right; it is red, solar, and masculine. There is some suggestion in the literature that when a yogi is female, the spiraling ascends in a direction opposite that of a male yogi. The ida and the pingala entwine as they ascend the energy field counterpart of the spinal cord, and they meet the sushumna in the energy field overlying a place between the eyebrows "in a triple knot." They then separate, the ida exiting through the left nostril, the pingala through the right nostril.

These major nadis are stimulated when the kundalini energy is aroused from its latent state with citta through controlled yogic practices. When kundalini is thus aroused, it is said to be like a fire that burns everything impure in its path. Its goal is to reach two chakras, one in the heart region and the other overlying the throat. The consuming fire or heat of kundalini is obtained by a spiritual transmutation of sexual energies into, for example, selfless love or devotion or compassion.[5]

Yoga is far removed from simple ecstasy. Its goal is *samadhi*, or illumination. This is the state of highest concentration that comes only after the yogi has disciplined his or her fantasies, emotions, mental restlessness, and physical body with its physiological functioning. In samadhi, not only does the yogi have complete mastery of his or her physical being, but he or she also has a profound and personal experience of the sacred. In describing the great yogi Milarepa, Evan-Wentz states the process graphically: "As the chemist experiments with the elements of matter, Milarepa experimented with the elements of consciousness."[6]

The raison d'être of yoga is the in-depth study of human consciousness. For this reason, I have often thought of Therapeutic Touch as a yoga of healing. Unlike Western thought, which recognizes only the brain and, more recently, possibly the immunological system, as seats of human consciousness, Indian thought considers the nonphysical chakras as centers of consciousness. The chakras are described as patterned vortices of energy whose centers are connected with the sushumna nadi.[7] These vortices act as centers of consciousness for such awarenesses as space-consciousness, inner movement, emotion, and other qualitative expressions of the psyche.[8]

There are several major and minor such vortices in a person's energy field. Seven of the major chakras and their relationship to the Therapeutic Touch process are discussed below. The best contemporary sources of information about the chakras are *The Chakras and the Human Energy Field*, by Karagulla and Kunz,[9] and *The Personal Aura*, by Kunz.[10]

Using the spinal cord as a reference, the lowermost chakra is called the *muladhara*. The prefix *mula* means "root," and the chakra is located in the energy field at the base of the spinal column between the anal orifice and the genital organs, at the site of the sacrococcygeal plexus of spinal nerves. It is here that kundalini is said to "sleep" in such a position that it blocks access to the prime nadi, the sushumna. Kundalini is related to forces deep within Earth, to the cohesive power of matter, to inertia, and to the sense of smell, and its energy is said to be the basis for the present evolutionary thrust of this planet.[11, 12]

The next chakra is the spleen chakra. It is not widely noted in the literature, but has been attested to in more recent times.[13] It is concerned with the specialization, subdivision, and distribution of prana, which is said to come from the sun and to be closely allied with the oxygen molecule. From the perspective of Western physiology, the function of the physical spleen is the regeneration of red blood cells. Red blood cells contain hemoglobin, a respiratory pigment whose function is to attach to oxygen molecules as they enter the lung tissue on inspiration and to distribute them to the body's cells. This is a necessity for the life process since human metabolism is mainly oxidative. The Indian view of the spleen chakra seems quite rational in light of this Western understanding. There are techniques in Therapeutic Touch for using this chakra to accelerate the healing process.

The next chakra up the spine is the *manipura* chakra, which is also called *nabhisthana*; *nabhi* means "umbilicus" and is a description of the area in the lumbar region where this chakra is found. This chakra is said to be related to the element fire, to the breath, to the sun, to the menstrual flow in women, to the sense of sight, and to the transformation of certain organic substances into psychic energies of the more sensuous emotions. There may be a correspondence with the current theory of psychosomatic ills. It is in this chakra's location that people under consistent high stress get peptic ulcers or spasmodic stomachaches as a result of pent-up anger, anxiety, or other such emotions. So certainly there is acknowledgment, if not agreement, with the Indian interpretation. Symptoms of stress respond very well to the use of certain Therapeutic Touch techniques with this chakra.

The *anahata* is the chakra that overlies the heart. It is the seat of prana, the life energy, and of the *jivatman*, the soul. It is related to the element air, to the sense of touch, to the force of nerves that send information throughout the body, and to the blood system.

In Western terms, it regulates respiration, the heart function, and the circulatory system via the sympathetic nervous system. The anahata chakra is also said to govern the plane of human realization. Since the central teaching of the Christ figure is that love, the "heart energy," is the ultimate basis for the fulfillment of human life, it may be that the full development of this chakra is the evolutionary goal of the present era.

At the laryngeal and pharyngeal nerves plexuses, where the head of the spinal cord and the medulla oblongata at the base of the brain join, is the *vishuddha*, or throat, chakra. It is the seat of *udana*, one of the five fires of sacrifice. It is also the site of the breath that is said to carry the soul to the head in the samadhi state of illumination. This site governs the conscious transformation of prana through mantric power, the power of controlled sound. The vishuddha chakra is related to the *akasha*—the continuum of consciousness, to the substrate of sound, and to the skin, through which we feel vibration.

The *ajna*, or "third eye," chakra between the eyebrows is in the cavernous plexus of nerves. It is at this site that the nadis—the sushumna, the ida, and the pingala—meet. *Ajna* means "to command" or "to order." This chakra is the seat of the cognitive and subtle senses of perception, and it functions in conjunction with the *sahasrara* chakra at the crown of the head.

Sahasrara means "thousand," for this crown chakra is represented symbolically by the thousand-petaled lotus. The lotus, although anchored in the waters of the Earth, has petals in a different medium, the air. So this chakra is considered to be the link between the personality of the space/time material world and the higher functions of the self. It is associated with the pituitary-pineal axis and is concerned with volition, acts of will, and altruism.

The Experience of Therapeutic Touch

The basis for this analysis of the Therapeutic Touch process so far has been the healing interaction of human energy fields from an abstract and theoretical perspective. However, what can be said about the living experiential knowledge that is involved in this most humane of human interactions? Experiential Exercise 11 sets up a structured situation for objectively examining the subtle cues picked up by the healer during the Therapeutic Touch experiences.

EXPERIENTIAL EXERCISE 11

The Human Barrier Game

Any even number of people can play this game. Each person chooses a partner, preferably a person not well known. Each couple then decides between themselves who will play the roles of healer and healee.

Each of the participants should have notepaper and a pen nearby. A chair is also needed for the healee. The chair is placed in such a manner that the healee can sit sideways on it, enabling the healer to reach the healee's back. The healer can either stand by the side of the healee or sit in another chair.

The Human Barrier Game is a three-part exercise. There is a pause after each part for both healer and healee to write their impressions in their journals.

Part I

1. Both the healer and healee take a moment to center.

2. The healer then does a full assessment of the healee's energy field. While maintaining a centered state of consciousness, the healee tries to become aware of the subtle interaction between his/her energy field and that of the healer.

3. At the end of the assessment, both healer and healee write their impressions in their journals. They do not exchange information until the end of the exercise.

Part II

1. Once again, both the healer and healee take a moment to center.

2. The healer then stands quietly at the healee's side while the healee mentally visualizes a strong barrier that effectively keeps out the intrusion of the healer's energy field and makes the healer unable to interact. The healee can use any method that comes to mind to create the visualized barrier.

3. When the healee feels that such a barrier is in place, he or she nods or otherwise signals to the healer.

4. The healer then does another assessment on the healee, noting particularly any differences in the healee's energy field from the first assessment.

5. When the healer is finished with the assessment, both the healer and the healee again note their impressions in their journals.

Part III

1. Once again, the healee and healer begin by centering.

2. The healee again sets up the visualized barrier and signals the healer when this is accomplished.

3. The healer does another assessment on the healee, noting the barrier. However, this time the healer attempts to break through the barrier using any technique learned in Therapeutic Touch practice that could do the job. Whether the healer can or cannot get through the barrier becomes evident within a few minutes. Both people should not persist in this portion of the exercise for more than three minutes.

4. Both the healer and healee again write up their impressions, answering the following questions:
   For the healer: In what ways did the healee's energy field

feel different once the barrier was in place? How did you break through the barrier? What techniques did you use? Do you think you succeeded? What gives you that impression?

For the healee: What was the barrier that you visualized? What did it feel like when the healer was trying to break through your barrier? Did the healer succeed?

5. After both the healer and healee have finished their notes, they report to the group, if they are doing this exercise with others, or discuss their findings with each other.

6. At the end of the discussion, the healer and healee change roles and repeat the exercise.

The Search for Ordering Principles

Several questions on the dynamics of illness and healing have presented themselves to me over the years. Why do some people get sick and not others? has been one such question. Its corollary has also perplexed me: Why do some people get well and not others? There has also been this strange paradox: Why do some people not get well and even die, yet while they live behave in a "healed" manner indicating they have found significant meaning, purpose, and satisfaction in their time on Earth? This apparent incongruity has led me to question whether there are logical ordering principles undergirding both Therapeutic Touch and the entire healing process. This is a quest I have continued to pursue, and it was within this context that I developed the Human Barrier Game.

The Human Barrier Game has turned out to be a very good source of qualitative data. This data indicates that a structured search for ordering principles foundational to the Therapeutic Touch process is feasible. Table I and Table II present a simple tabulation of random experiences of persons who have played the Human Barrier Game.

TABLE I

Close Relationships Between Healees' Visualizations of Their Barriers and Healers' Impressions of the Barriers in a Random Group Playing the Human Barrier Game

HEALEE'S VISUALIZATION OF BARRIER	HEALER'S IMPRESSION OF BARRIER
Bubble of energy	Balloon
Clear shell	"I felt nothing."
Plexiglas	Cool, impenetrable
Steel door	Hard, smooth
Thick concrete wall	"I couldn't get close."
Walnut shell	Rippled surface
"I pulled my field over me and hid."	"I smoothed out her energy field, sort of pulling it inside-out, and grounded her."
"I felt strain at my throat [from maintaining the barrier] and gritted my teeth."	"I felt as if she had stopped radiating."
"I went someplace else and took myself away."	"I felt nothing from her, nothing at all."
"I was sitting in a barrel that extended to my eyes."	"I got in through the back of her neck, at about the level of her eyes."
Used King Arthur's armor: "It took a lot of work to maintain the barrier. . . . I realized that my back was unprotected."	"The air over his body felt different. He was breathing differently, holding something in. The holding area was in the back of his neck."
Closed in and protected by porcupine quills	"It was easy to get in, once he let go and relaxed."
"I put myself into the freezer in my garage."	"I cut through the barrier, getting a little heat, a strong energy flow going."

"I was in the chorus line of the Rockettes, and I kept kicking her out rhythmically."

"I overextended and solidified my energy field all around until I felt crystallized."

"I felt as though her energy field was bobbing up and down."

"He was in a strong chamber that had a negative or a different environment so that everything was tight, hard, and sharp-edged."

TABLE II

Visualized Protective Barriers, Treatment of Barriers with Therapeutic Touch Techniques, and Comments of Participants During the Human Barrier Game

BARRIER	TREATMENT	COMMENTS
Emotion		
Anger	Unruffling to relax healee	Healee A: "I felt the anger slip away." Healee B: "I kept losing the image." Healee C: "I feel balanced again."
Hostility	Touch	Healee A: "I pushed my energy field out, away from myself. The touch broke through my resolve." Healer A: "I just reached in where he was closed off." Healee B: "I pulled everything in, like a turtle that is retreating into his shell. I had to work hard to keep her out." Healer B: "I felt that I could not get all the way through the barrier, which was very hard and resistant." Healee C: "It really tired me to keep up the barrier." Healer C: "I wanted to support her."
	Love	Healee: "I felt a tugging at my heart. It felt so nice that I had to let go."

		Healer: "I had to expend so much energy to engage the barrier. Then, all of a sudden, this sense of compassion flooded over me and broke it down."
Rage	Love	Healee A: "I absolutely engulfed myself in a sense of rage, but in a short while I felt nothing, just quiet. Maybe that is what is called *peace*." Healee B: "I felt exhausted by the great amount of energy it took to maintain the rage. Then I felt washed by this wave of rosy light and felt refreshed and cool."
	Touch	Healee: "In my rage, I felt as if everything was black and chaotic and nobody could find me. But as soon as she touched me, she went right in. I was astonished at how fast she went through my barrier."
Tensed muscles "I cut off my feelings."	Relaxation response, deep caring	Healee: "I was not going to reveal myself, but it was very difficult work. Then I just had to let go. I guess I wanted to let go." Healer: "It was clear to me that I was working with two different people.

Structures

Barbed wire or projectiles	Deep penetration of energy	Healee A: "It was very hard work to keep up the barrier." Healer A: "I just poka-tru!" Healee B: "The metal spears and daggers turned to soft putty."
Block of ice	Relaxation response, love	Healee A: "The ice just melted." Healee B: "I felt his energy come through like waves of warmth, and it opened up my heart."

		Healer B: "It was not a very pleasant experience, but there was nothing else I could do, so I offered love."
		Healee C: "I just thought: She's going to hurt me. I'm not going to feel."
		Healer C: "I didn't think that blasting him with energy would work. He wasn't even there."
Cement block	Heart chakra connection	Healee A: "When her energy hit my chest, I felt her energy move my energy."
		Healer A: "The barrier was so cold and inhuman that I felt compassion and love."
		Healee B: "She got to me through the heart."
		Healer B: "I centered more deeply and used my heart chakra."
	Touch	Healee: "Once he touched me, I didn't feel as secure as I had thought I was."
		Healer: "I also talked to the area [barrier] in my mind."
Cloak of armor	Deep penetration of energy	Healee: "Then I realized that it didn't cover my neck or feet, and I felt an ache in my forehead and feet."
		Healer: "I got in through the feet— they were the most vulnerable."
Cocoon	Relaxation response	Healee: "It was a lot of work. I had to keep putting more layers on."
		Healer: "I felt the hard toughness of her barrier."
Electric circuit board	Love and compassion	Healee: "Suddenly I felt myself saying, 'No!' but the struts broke and I couldn't hold the circuit."

Glassy, cool surface	Projected heat from heart chakra	**Healee:** "My heart area got warm, and the barrier melted." **Healer:** "Meanwhile, I talked to her in my head."
Intense cold	Deep projection of energy	**Healer:** "This rhythm in her field slowed and got sluggish, so I energized her at the adrenals until I felt the energy flow smoothly again."
Lead shield	Touch	**Healee:** "I felt that if she touched me, placed a hand on me, I would shatter. She did, and the barrier split apart."
Man-eating sharks	Heart chakra connection	**Healee:** "The sharks turned into angels." **Healer:** "She felt as though she were afraid, and I wanted to protect her."
Metal fortress	Projected cool energy	**Healee:** "I felt the energy force pushing me backward. I had to struggle to maintain my balance." **Healer:** "The tingling feeling changed to heat to keep me out, so I just 'cooled' it."
Rigid boundary	Love	**Healee:** "I found that I wanted to open the boundary. It was difficult to resist." **Healer:** "It was a very tough barrier, so I smiled sweetly and got in through the level of the heart and throat chakras."
	Gentle energy projection	**Healer:** "I 'saw' a heavy, impenetrable concrete tube around her, but it did not go all the way down to her feet. So I gently projected energy there, and it got through."

Stone	Deep caring	Healee A: "It was difficult to maintain the barrier. I felt close to tears." Healee B: "I tried to go someplace else. The love was too much."
Triple bubble	Unruffling	Healer: "There were so many layers that I felt that only by unruffling her energy field would I get through."
Saran Wrap	Unruffling	Healer: "It was slippery, strange. I felt that I got through the only chink in her shiny armor."
Ziploc bag	Heart chakra connection	Healee: "I felt this warm, gentle pressure. I was glad to get out! I felt as if I had been frozen alive."

Comments on the Human Barrier Game

These tables are only rough sketches of actual Therapeutic Touch interactions. However, they do indicate that the Human Barrier Game is a useful tool for understanding the patterns of thought and symbolic images with which people protect themselves. The tables also provide some insight into how the healing process is therapeutic for persons who seek to isolate themselves in a manner that may not be in their best interest. Finally, they support the reality of the cues in the healee's energy field and therefore provide some substantiation for the existence of the "Emperor's Clothes."

A fully structured study has yet to be done. Indeed, I am presenting this material in the hope of stimulating interest in such a study. However, there are a few generalizations that can be made from the present data. One is that it took a tremendous exertion of energy for the healees to maintain their visualizations of the barriers. They felt disconnected by the barriers and lost their sense of being grounded. They found it particularly difficult to resist the healers' projections of love, gentleness, or deep caring, and physical touch was very powerful in reaching them.

To the healers, the barriers frequently felt "flat," "empty," or "like vacuums." Sometimes the healers "couldn't find" the healees' energy flows, or there was little or no interchange of energies. In other instances, the healers could assess the healees' energy fields using either specific cues or "resonance," through which the healers' hands naturally gravitated to the right places or the healers found the healees' vulnerable sites using an incontestable intuitive sense.

In conclusion, the Human Barrier Game indicates that unfettered human energy is flow, and that visualization bolstered by intentionality can significantly affect this flow. Also, the game points out that it is possible to identify the nature and quality of another person's visualizations using a kind of psychic pattern-recognition ability to which everyone is heir. Finally, it is apparent from this exercise that love is an irresistible and mysterious energy.

Time

Other generalizations that have maintained their validity and reliability over the two decades Dora Kunz and I have developed Therapeutic Touch are also intriguing and worthy of further study. One such generalization concerns time. In Therapeutic Touch, time—as expressed by the timing of events in the healing process—is different from linear, clock time. The Therapeutic Touch process significantly accelerates positive changes in symptomatology and speeds recuperation beyond expectation. In a study on increases in blood components during the laying-on of hands[14] that was later replicated using the Therapeutic Touch process,[15] healees' hemoglobin levels and hematocrit values changed very quickly. In one subset of patients who had severe anemias, the increase in blood components was significant within two hours.[16]

In clinical studies, healees have exhibited a full relaxation response in two to four minutes. In studies on women with Raynaud's disease, a severe disturbance of the circulation in the extremities, symptoms have disappeared in three to four minutes, with a return of natural coloration and feeling to the extremities. In supervised clinical studies on paralytic ileus, which may occur following surgical operations on the gastrointestinal tract, there has been consistent evidence of very rapid autonomic nervous system response. The same has been true with studies on problems of the smooth muscle tissues of the genitourinary tract. As previously noted, the body's fluid and electrolyte balance is also very sensitive to Therapeutic Touch, exhibited by the unusually rapid reduction of persistent dependent edema following Therapeutic Touch.

Timing is also a significant factor in two other ways in the practice of Therapeutic Touch. First, if Therapeutic Touch is implemented early in amenable disease processes, symptoms are frequently significantly ameliorated or eradicated. However, if Therapeutic Touch is used late in the disease process, symptoms may persist, although the patient may undergo an unexpected and personally meaningful psychological transformation. Second, it has been repeatedly demonstrated that two persons doing Therapeutic Touch to the same healee must rhythmically mesh their efforts to rebalance the healee's energies. Otherwise, the healee may experience ill effects such as nausea, dizziness, or irritability. Also, Therapeutic Touch has been successfully used for problems related to natural rhythms of the body. These include menstrual dysfunctions, problems during pregnancy, and repetitive dysfunctional emotional states such as manic depression, all of which are cyclic phenomena.

Intensity

Another consistently important variable is the intensity with which Therapeutic Touch is practiced. It has already been mentioned that it is possible for the healee to overdose on energy when Therapeutic Touch is overly prolonged and sufficient attention is not paid by the practitioner to the healee's sensitivity to the process. The signs of overdose to watch for in the healee bear repeating: increasing restlessness leading to heightened irritability, anxiety, hostility, or even pain if the intervention is heedlessly continued. These responses are so contrary to the original purpose of the healing practice that you, as the healer, are cautioned to be thoughtfully conservative rather than impulsive in your energetic interactions.

A simple general rule to observe is the following: the sicker the healee, the gentler you should be in performing Therapeutic Touch and the shorter the period should be during which you intervene. This is particularly wise when working with little children, persons with brain injury, or healees about whom little is known.

System Sensitivity

With respect to the fundamental ordering principles of the Therapeutic Touch process, it is important to keep in mind the high sensitivity of certain body systems. As mentioned before, these include the autonomic nervous system, the lymphatic system, the circulatory system, and portions of the endocrine system such as the thyroid gland, the adrenal glands, and the endocrine glands involved in pregnancy, menses, and the climacteric. Such sensitivity is apparent in the unexpectedly good results of Therapeutic Touch with persons experiencing certain severe psychological disorders such as manic depression, catatonia, and extreme hyperactivity.

Centers of Consciousness

The assessment flow sheet clearly indicates that the Therapeutic Touch dynamic is related to cognitive factors of the healer such as memory, judgment, evaluation, and decision making, as well as cue-specific information that wells up from the unconscious and through the intuition of the healer. When specific centers of consciousness, the chakras, are used in Therapeutic Touch, predictable effects occur. For instance, in Experiential Exercise 8, the area of the body near which the hands are placed, over the adrenals, is essentially the manipura, or the solar plexus, chakra.

As noted previously, work with the solar plexus chakra is particularly helpful for energizing persons suffering from fatigue and invariably helps everyone on whom the work is done. From the Indian perspective, the solar plexus chakra energizes a large number of important organs, including the adrenals, pancreas, liver, stomach, and intestinal tract. This is why Therapeutic Touch, when used in the region of this chakra, is so beneficial to so many people, especially in these stress-laden times. Many parts of the body affected by stress are reached through the solar plexus.

Similarly, work over the anahata, or heart chakra, sensitizes the healee to the power of contactual touch, which has a close connection with deep caring—an emotion often characterized as "coming from the heart." There are ways to use the heart chakra in the Therapeutic Touch interaction with those in emergencies or other crisis situations, as noted in chapter 5. This chakra is also related to the blood system, and Therapeutic Touch at this site is very effective for persons with cardiac arrhythmias and hypertension.

On the basis of impressions strengthened by years of Therapeutic Touch practice, I feel that the vishudda, or throat chakra, which is concerned with aspiration and compassion, is stimulated in persons who practice Therapeutic Touch. In addition, I feel that persons engaged in healing as a lifestyle may gain access to the higher, or finer, chakras—the ajna and sahasrara chakras—via consistent acts of intentionality and an altruism fired by compassion and selfless love. Such behavior indicates a personal intention to control citta, the psyche's willful function of impetuousness, fantasy, and impatience. It also indicates an intention to replace this function with thoughtful reflection and a concentration empowered by focus and anchored to reality.

It is instructive to observe how habitual involvement in the act of centering alters your worldview in important ways. Characteristic of this state of consciousness are an implicit sense of timelessness and a clear recognition that there are no "boundaries" in the realm of the mind. Opportunity for the redirection of your own personality thereby becomes possible when the active engagement of yourself in the daily activity of living becomes a conscious, mindful act. In fact, the healing act that you perform for yourself with the committed engagement of Therapeutic Touch practice is the development of your ability to change, for change is the handmaiden of healing.

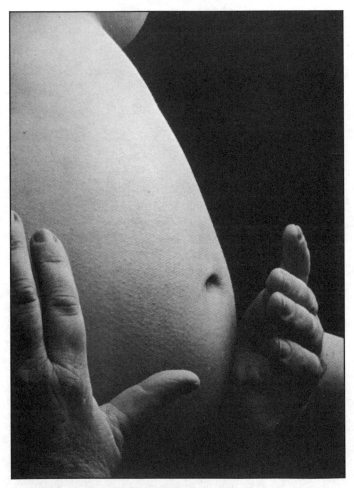

FIGURE 11. Therapeutic Touch and the Pregnant Mother

Chapter 5

SPECIFIC USES
OF THERAPEUTIC TOUCH

Before you make a commitment to Therapeutic Touch practice, it is important that you understand the difference between the concept of *curing* and the concept of *healing* so that the context of the Therapeutic Touch process is clear. The word *cure* comes from Latin and connotes "to care for." Early in the history of the Christian church, the *curate* was concerned with caring for the soul. In more recent times, the term *cure* has come to be associated with a system or particular method of medical treatment. The phrase "to be cured for five years," for instance, could be interpreted as meaning that under a specific system of treatment the patient is expected to live for five years.

On the contrary, the term *heal* comes from the Middle English word *helen*, "to make whole" or "to care about" (rather than to care *for*) the whole or total individual. The term *heal* therefore has to do with how one thinks of oneself and others—with one's worldview or personal philosophy. Consequently, healing is concerned with the quality of life across its entire spectrum. It is concerned with the transformation of personality and the transcendence of life conditions, and the fostering of this personal growth in the healee is the ultimate goal of the Therapeutic Touch practitioner.

Both transformation and transcendence are subjective, of course. Nevertheless, a leading tenet of psychoneuroimmunology, one of the most promising interdisciplinary approaches to disease processes that continue to escape understanding, is that subjective mood profoundly affects the neuropeptides stationed throughout the body. The importance of this is made apparent by the fact that neuropeptides affect the functioning of endorphins and enkephalins. These latter not only alleviate pain but also actively promote a sense of well-being.

An example of the effects of Therapeutic Touch on persons with severe spinal cord injuries might clarify this. In instances of transverse myelitis, in which the spinal cord has been cut and the persons are paralyzed from the site of the lesion down, Therapeutic Touch does not cause the parts of the spinal cord to grow together or remove the paralysis. However, after receiving Therapeutic Touch, these persons report a greater sense of vitality, more vigor in their daily activities, and an uplifted psychological outlook on life. They report that they act in a more integrated and focused manner in day-to-day problem solving and have an increased sense of self-esteem. I would call this a successful healing, even though it is not a cure.

Moreover—and I do admit that this is strange and difficult to account for—many of these persons report that, although they have neither sensory nor motor abilities below the lesion, they can "feel" the person doing Therapeutic Touch to them, even in their extremities. At a large rehabilitation center on the East Coast, I had an opportunity to test these claims in a pilot study with a small sample of five young men, each with a transected spinal cord. The men were blindfolded and then a nurse was brought in whom none of them knew. Each man was tested individually as the nurse did Therapeutic Touch to his energy field, without making contact with his skin. Not only did each of the five men report feeling the Therapeutic Touch interaction, but four of them, still blindfolded, could tell exactly where the nurse's hands were in their energy fields during the Therapeutic Touch interaction.

The healing process itself is awesome to witness. It has an elegant beauty and indescribable grace in its harmonic regularity and specificity. The healing of a wound, say a small but deep cut on the hand, is remarkable. Under normal circumstances it often heals without an observable scar or any other indication that anything once marred the intact tissue. However, the exquisite nature of this dynamic healing process is clearly revealed by microscopy. Observed from this enlarged perspective, it is clear that the healing process involves several levels of organization. The materials for seven different cellular layers are biochemically routed, each to its appropriate place on the molecular space lattice, as the wounded tissues mend and become functional again.

As this remarkable natural healing process is studied at greater magnification, certain less obvious, although equally significant processes are also dynamically engaged. Synchronization is one such process. At the molecular level, several biochemical substances must be brought into specific, precise, spatial relationships with each other on a schedule that is exactly timed. Yet, even as this magical happening is observed and marveled upon, it presents a provocative and profound question: Who, or perhaps, what, is the master choreographer of these finely tuned microstrategies that bind together the pieces of the healing act?

Eons of time have yet to release the secret of these barely comprehensible questions. Nevertheless, the spectrum of wonder can be further extended: how can healing be so selective that it can inhibit the chaotic growth of tissues that are malignant and yet vigorously stimulate the precise growth of diverse, new, healthy tissues in wound healing? In the end, we must admit the obvious: healing is, indeed, a profound mystery.

How can this mystery be understood? Perhaps understanding is too much to expect. However, I do think that over time an appreciation of these abstruse happenings can seep into conscious awareness in the course of centering during the Therapeutic Touch process. The act of centering has as its goal the extension of consciousness into the profound quietude characteristic of the deep self. It is the appreciation of a nonverbal reality that in fact guides the process.

This appreciation occurs most naturally in the rebalancing phase of Therapeutic Touch. During the attempt to bring the healee's energies into a state of harmonic balance, the underlying, intelligent concentration of forces at work in the healing process is the most impressive. As the rebalancing of the healee's energies proceeds, it is apparent that not only is the healthy human energy field symmetrically aligned and in a state of dynamic equipoise, but all of its component factors are elegantly integrated and superbly synchronized in the interest of maintaining that delicate balance we call life.

This nonverbal reality is beyond our human language to express, beyond our logic to understand, and beyond our cultural mores to structure. Therefore, it can act as a bridge for the transpersonal,[1] and when it does, the healing act becomes creative. As the exploration of the deep self continues, you learn to maintain a keen sense of mindfulness during the healing interaction. Out of this state of consciousness may flow unsought an effortless awareness of the unitive relationship between yourself and the healee. On occasion, this process will manifest a glimpse of the underlying reasons for the healee's illness.

There are, of course, many mountains that you as the healer cannot climb—much that is beyond your reach. However, if you can learn to stay in this powerful state of consciousness, you will find, with few exceptions, that the deeper you are able to go into awareness, the easier it will be for you to reach and help the ill person.

How Therapeutic Touch Has Been Used

Recently, I spent an entire day in the clinic of a hospital where Therapeutic Touch is practiced. My caseload schedule for that particular day is reproduced below.

TIME	NAME	DIAGNOSIS
8:30 a.m.	Frank	Low back and left shoulder pain
9:15	Hilda	Rheumatoid arthritis
10:00	Marion	Postabdominal surgery
10:45	Phoebe	Cancer of the uterus
11:30	Thelma	Cancer of the breast (left)

lunch	George	Panic attack (emergency consult)
1:00 p.m.	Jenny	Temporomandibular joint pain
1:45	Bobbie (4 years old)	HIV+
	Hazel (2½ years old)	HIV+
2:30	Connie	Multiple sclerosis
3:15	Martin	Peptic ulcer

This is an unusually wide range of ailments for one modality to attempt to alleviate. However, there were some commonalties in the treatments of several pairs of the healees: Frank and Hilda, Phoebe and Thelma, and the two children, Bobbie and Hazel, who had been exposed to AIDS since birth. Nevertheless, each treatment had to be individualized, for there are many different factors that can predispose a person to illness, and the healer must seek the underlying problem in each instance. A few examples of the causes of illness are foods that trigger allergic reactions, distraught emotions and prolonged stress, iatrogenic illnesses from side reactions to medications, exposure to very-low-frequency radiation when working near electronic equipment, and secondary reactions to illnesses or organic damage.

Therapeutic Touch primarily works with the symptoms elicited during illness. This chapter contains accounts of specific uses of Therapeutic Touch. However, it is important that you not regard this information as prescriptive, since each situation you face will present unique features for you to deal with.

I will also restate that the only concern of Therapeutic Touch is with human energies. Therefore, medical diagnoses per se are not necessarily relevant to its use. Nevertheless, since most illnesses are widely known by terms that come out of the diagnostic framework, they have been retained in the following discussions. It is assumed that you will bring to the situations you encounter in your own life all that you have learned thus far. It is evident to those of you who have begun to use Therapeutic Touch that neither its phases nor the situations in which it is used are time bound.

Thus, it is useless to prescribe Therapeutic Touch in recipe fashion.

In the following discussions, I share ways that I have used Therapeutic Touch in my own practice and research, but the essence of the Therapeutic Touch interaction involves you as the practitioner consciously using your innermost resources in the interest of helping another being who is in need. Therefore, the decision about how to help a healee relies strongly on your personal judgment and the clarity of interpretation of thoughts that well up from your centered focus to your deep self. While there are certain commonalities to most problems of human energy imbalance, it is the individual, in as much totality as can be comprehended, who is the context of the Therapeutic Touch interaction.

The situations discussed below were chosen because they include a wide range of symptoms—that is, patterns of human energy dysfunction—many of which are also encountered in other illnesses. For example, the information on the dissipation of pain contained in the section on pregnancy can be used in other situations involving pain. And the information on the use of Therapeutic Touch to help persons undergoing chemotherapy, which is in the section on persons who are HIV+, can be applied to persons undergoing chemotherapy for other reasons.

It is important to firmly grasp that you, as the healer, are accepting the responsibility of using Therapeutic Touch in a conscious and judicious manner. It is you who makes the decisions about the Therapeutic Touch interactions, you who judges when it is appropriate to initiate the Therapeutic Touch process, you who decides what to do about the healee's problem, and you who decides when to terminate the interaction. Therefore, be there for the person in need—totally.

Pregnancy

Interest in using Therapeutic Touch during pregnancy grew out of a research study of mine that was funded by the United States Public Health Service in 1983 and 1984.[2] The premise of the study was that a husband, in doing Therapeutic Touch to his wife during pregnancy, would significantly deepen his sensitivity to and awareness of both the mother and the growing fetus. As a consequence, a concerned and satisfying relationship of mutual deep caring would develop within the family. This turned out to be the case.

Perhaps the most rewarding aspect of this study was the clear recognition by the parents that we do not stop at our skins. This realization opened the way for the husband to see that if there were no real boundaries or cutoff points to his energy field, this was also true for his wife and child. This insight led to increased sensitivity to each individual within the family and to the family as a whole.

Since this study was reported in 1984, it has been competently replicated, and the results have been shown to be reliable. Therapeutic Touch has been integrated into the practices of registered midwives, Lamaze teachers, and nurses, and it has been taught by them to many pregnant couples in the United States and Canada, usually during the seventh to ninth months of gestation.

After the study, many persons who had taken part in it reported to me that they had continued to use Therapeutic Touch in their everyday lives. At first, they used Therapeutic Touch for postnatal problems such as the healing of the episiotomy and sore breasts. Then, as the family members took up their lives at home, it became natural for them to use Therapeutic Touch for common ailments such as colds, coughs, headaches, indigestion, general stress reduction, and emotional support.

At this writing, there is general agreement that the strength garnered from the increased sensitivity to and understanding of other family members extended itself to everyday involvement in outside affairs. Other poststudy findings include the following:

- Therapeutic Touch practice created close bonds within the family and gave family members a sense of increased inner strength to meet unexpected contingencies from a deeper, shared perspective.

- Additional family members were intrigued by the effects of Therapeutic Touch and also wanted to be involved in its practice.

- Therapeutic Touch opened participants to the recognition of their own psychic potentials, which they then used actively and creatively in their daily relationships.

- From a purely pragmatic point of view, the act of centering allowed the husband, who was most often the sole breadwinner, to shift his consciousness from the demanding, ego-centered personal involvement sparked by the highly competitive atmosphere of the business marketplace to a broader, humanitarian frame of reference.

- In some families, it became a practice several times a week for the wife to do Therapeutic Touch to her husband when he came home from work, and vice versa. Working particularly over the kidney-adrenal and heart regions effected a rapid relaxation response. This relaxation response marked the release of personal nervous energies that had been used in an overly long, continuous fashion, and indicated a refreshing shift to more unbounded, natural energies.

- The continued practice of Therapeutic Touch, particularly its centering or meditative aspect, helped the wife to keep in touch with her interior life. In so doing, she became very sensitive to, and developed a growing relationship with, the living being within herself during the pregnancy. This inner awareness also served to heighten the mother's recognition of warning psychophysiological signals about her health or that of the growing fetus, when they arose. Later, after the birth, the mother experienced special times of awakening to her child's infanthood.

- The wives also said that centering, which many continued to do throughout their pregnancies, helped them shift their perspectives on life, for through the Therapeutic Touch experience they realized the bona fide reality of human energies. During pregnancy, many of the women spent time every day trying to access and understand how these energies operated within themselves. Their goal was to learn how to consciously assist these dynamical energies to work for themselves and their growing families.

Under normal conditions of pregnancy, you would primarily use Therapeutic Touch to elicit a relaxation response, promote rest and sleep, and reduce discomfort. Lamaze techniques to prepare for the delivery work very well in conjunction with Therapeutic Touch practices.

Labor and Delivery

Birth is a wondrous natural event, but most of us are so divorced from the natural that it is awesome to observe the autonomous, persistent, and progressive march of events that occurs once birthing begins. Under normal conditions, nature needs little help to birth her young. Therefore, the major role of the father of the child or his surrogate is to be intelligently helpful and supportive, and to remain relaxed but aware of the unfolding process.

The following Therapeutic Touch techniques can assist the mother in the labor and delivery process. These suggestions assume that the birth process is normal and that the birthing is under the supervision of a competent and knowledgeable person.

- At the onset of labor, the mother can help herself by first centering and then unruffling her own energy field in a downward and outward direction. Starting at the upper abdomen where it overlies the fundus (within which lies the child), and with the palms of her hands turned outward, she should direct any congestion outward from the inner, more central part of her energy field, at about the level of her breastbone, toward the periphery of her energy field. It is particularly useful if she exhales at the same time. Exercises in imagery are also helpful adjuncts at this point.

- The father of the child can help the mother's efforts by putting his hand chakras over the mother's heart and conveying love and support.

- Should the contractions be uncomfortable, the father can unruffle the mother's energy field in an unhurried, rhythmic fashion.

- The father can also assist the flow of energy down the mother's legs and out the natural exit of the foot chakras.

- In addition, the father can support the mother's efforts by placing his hand chakras over her kidney-adrenal area and, without strain, directing his (normally excess) energy flows to her. He is often most comfortable and comforting doing this while sitting behind her on the bed or other birthing place. In this posture, he can use the trunk of his body to physically support the mother while he places his hand chakras over her kidney-adrenal area. As previously noted, this directing of energies can be facilitated if it is done with a sense of intentionality on the exhalation of breath. A light massage of the mother's lower back also can be incorporated.

- As with pregnancy, these Therapeutic Touch skills can be coupled with Lamaze techniques.

All comfort measures, of course, should be included with these Therapeutic Touch processes. Because of the nature of the situation, they can have irreplaceable symbolic as well as practical value as indications of deep caring. Once the delivery of the child has begun, nature sets up her own scenario that, like all else concerned with the pregnancy, has a rhythm of its own. The drama is played out in "real time," and contingencies are met when, and if, they arise.

Postnatal Treatment

After a child is born, there are many ways that Therapeutic Touch can be helpful:

- If the mother has had an episiotomy or a Caesarean section, either she or her husband or other intimate person can do Therapeutic Touch to the wounded area to ease the discomfort and accelerate the healing process.

- Therapeutic Touch is very helpful if the baby is colicky or has a gas bubble it cannot expel. If you are the healer, gently hold the child against your shoulder and use your other hand to unruffle and then soothe the child's energy field. This usually displaces the bubble quite rapidly, within a minute or so.

- If the baby is irritable or crying, and if upon examination there appears to be no external problem such as an opened pin or other sharp object causing the baby to cry, then place the baby against your body, with its head upon your shoulder. Walk or sit and rock the baby, and do Therapeutic Touch to it. After a few minutes, the baby will respond characteristically: quite suddenly, the child will stop crying, open its eyes wide, and concentrate its gaze on you with a surprised look on its face. It will then lay its head on your shoulder and fall asleep—accompanied frequently by a loud, clearly enunciated, and resounding burp!

Pain

The experience of pain is not easily forgotten. Sometimes the memory is so strong that, as it lingers, it brings in its train vivid, emotion-bound recollections. The intensity of this persistent recall may provoke severe psychophysiological consequences as the thought of the pain or the fear of its recurrence perseveres.

If the pain can be alleviated, or if it ceases, there is a release of attention from this exclusive focus on the self and a reawakening to the presence of other people and experiences. This reprieve from reverberating, fear-shrouded, frustrating torment allows the experiencer to be vivified and to join the world again. This joy can be felt and quickly reciprocated by sensitive family members and friends who have been empathically experiencing the anguish of the sufferer, as well as their own grief.

To yourself as the Therapeutic Touch assessor, pain usually feels either like an area of turgid stasis or congestion in the healee's energy field or like a confusing jumble of conflicting energy levels. If the pain is prolonged or beyond the healee's level of endurance, the natural rhythmicity and internal dynamics of the healee's solar plexus chakra may be adversely affected.

As your hand chakras seek out cues to the energy imbalances, you may empathically pick up these powerful asynchronous effects. Your hands might actually feel the pain, or the subsequent nausea or fear. If you are able to maintain your own center of consciousness, you will quickly recognize that the pain or fear is not your own and will be able to go on with the business of helping the healee with his or her problem. However, if you overidentify with the situation and lose your original sense of intentionality, you stand a good chance of becoming part of the problem.

Clinically, Therapeutic Touch has been effective in alleviating or eradicating pain arising out of a large number of circumstances, and you as the Therapeutic Touch practitioner do not have to be very expert to help relieve a healee's pain. Following is a treatment routine that works very well:

1. After centering yourself, recall the wavelength of energy that you associate with the color blue. Sense this energy level as you would sense your body's tone; that is, sense it in your energy field as you would sense a state of calmness or quietude.

2. Fully experience the blueness for several moments.

3. Then, slowly project this blue energy as you gently

unruffle the healee's energy field around the painful site. Starting at or near the site, move the congested energy toward the periphery of the healee's energy field, where it will disperse and dissipate. It is important to keep your movements gentle, rhythmic, and sensitive to any change in the energy field.

4. Work over the healee's solar plexus, using the blue energy to quiet the healee's emotional reaction to the stress of the unpleasant experience of pain.

5. Do not prolong the rebalancing beyond twenty to twenty-five minutes. By then the pain will have lessened if it is amenable to Therapeutic Touch, and the healee will be experiencing a relaxation response.

6. After the treatment, have the healee lie down in a comfortable position and cover him or her with a light blanket. If the healee falls asleep and circumstances permit, allow him or her plenty of time to awaken naturally.

7. When the healee awakens, give him or her some imagery exercises as homework. Dora Kunz suggests having the healee imagine being by a beautiful seashore, watching the waves and imagining that the pain is reducing and receding with the waves as the tide ebbs.

Dora Kunz also suggests that if the healee can feel free of pain for even such a minimal amount of time as two minutes, the exercise can help to break the repetitive patterning of the pain. However, if the healee continues to feel pain, she suggests that you withdraw your hands from the healee's energy field and use other pain-reduction measures.

In their analysis of acupuncture, Chanes and Barber noted that a reduction in pain can be due to various psychological variables:[3]

- lowered anxiety level
- strong belief in the treatment's effectiveness

- special preparation and indoctrination before the treatment
- distraction of attention to pain
- the use of drugs

If the pain is protracted after the use of Therapeutic Touch, I would suggest referral to another source that can help.

Premenstrual Syndrome (PMS)

Premenstrual syndrome affects an estimated twenty-seven million women in the United States, which is about 40 percent of all women in this country. It can occur only occasionally, or it can occur repeatedly from menarche, which marks the initial onset of the menstrual cycle, to menopause, its cessation. Symptomatology may vary from woman to woman, and may differ in intensity from one cycle to the next in the same person. The following symptoms of PMS frequently occur, individually or multiply:

• mood changes	• neuroendocrinal system changes
• behavioral fluctuations	• general water retention
• irritability	• abdominal bloating
• depression	• breast engorgement
• anxiety	• lethargy
• impaired concentration	• fatigue
• headache	• food cravings

It is authoritatively stated that there are 150 additional symptoms. Strangely, although PMS is extremely complicated, it is not very difficult to relieve with Therapeutic Touch. It is treated symptomatically; that is, you can use Therapeutic Touch practices selectively for whatever a woman says is her presenting problem. I use a number of Therapeutic Touch techniques in trying to help her. Assuming that there are no gross organic abnormalities such as an inverted uterus, I use Therapeutic Touch in the following ways, based on a categorization of PMS symptoms.

Irritability and Anxiety

With problems of irritability, there is an energy overload whose patterning has gone awry. Consequently, the healee has become emotionally sensitive. After centering yourself:

- Rhythmically and gently unruffle the healee's energy field to help her release the pent-up congestion and to stimulate a controlled energy flow. Initially, spend only a few minutes on this unruffling.

- Then go on to stabilize her solar plexus chakra and heart chakra, using the energy of blue.

- Intersperse this chakra work with some gentle unruffling, working toward the goal of rebalancing the healee's whole system.

- To assist in this process, facilitate the energy flows in her field by directing them to and through the foot chakras as well as to the periphery of her energy field, where they will disperse.

- Take advantage of the healee's consequent relaxation response by having her lie down in a comfortable place that has good ventilation and, preferably, fresh air. See that she has a light blanket, and let her rest quietly.

As demonstrated in several formal studies, anxiety is very sensitive to Therapeutic Touch.[4-7] There are several different types of anxiety, but the predominant cause of all of them is stress. Anxiety is a feeling of apprehension and dread that may result in a prolonged state of fear. Awareness may be blocked by defense mechanisms, and many physical symptoms may emerge: tachycardia, dyspnea, tremors, excessive perspiration, nausea, muscular tension, restlessness, and breath-holding that may result in lightheadedness.

In your Therapeutic Touch assessment, you may feel the effects of this prolonged tension in the healee's overstrained energy field, together with a sense of dysrhythmia. Use Therapeutic Touch with an anxious person in a way similar to how you would use it for an irritable person. However, in addition:

- Help the throat chakra to stabilize and try to evoke a relaxation response as you use Therapeutic Touch over the solar plexus and heart chakras.

- Because prolonged anxiety easily feeds psychosomatic illnesses, refer the woman to someone who can help her lead a more balanced lifestyle through such techniques as yoga, meditation, imagery, and/or psychotherapy.

- Both shiatsu and acupressure have much to offer the woman with PMS. Therefore, you can either interface these techniques into your Therapeutic Touch practice or refer the healee to a competent shiatsu or acupressure practitioner. Then work in a congenial relationship with these practitioners for the well-being of the healee.

Lethargy, Fatigue, and Depression

In the following discussion, it is assumed that these signs do not mask deep psychological trauma.

Lethargy is marked by drowsiness, somnolence, or sluggish stupor. To you as the Therapeutic Touch assessor, the healee's energy field feels characteristic of a person who has an inability to absorb energy. This is coupled with indications of toxicity. For these reasons:

- The sites of choice for Therapeutic Touch are over the spleen chakra, to stimulate the pranic intake, and over the liver, to work on the toxicity. In practice, it feels as though there is an active but subtle energy flow between the splenic chakra and the liver, so it is good to work these two sites together. Be careful to use slow, gentle, rhythmic

movements and to frequently reassess the healee's
energy field.

- In addition, use Therapeutic Touch over the kidney-
adrenal area, at the site of the solar-plexus chakra complex, to encourage a stronger energy flow through the
system.

- Unruffle the healee's energy field to stimulate its functioning, and facilitate energized flows to and through the foot
chakras.

- As in all Therapeutic Touch practices, have the healee lie
down for ten to fifteen minutes after the treatment to give
her system an opportunity to absorb and receive optimal
benefit from the more efficient energy level.

Tiredness, lassitude, and weariness resulting from overexer-
tion or prolonged stress frequently accompany women who have
no choice (or recognize no choice) but to work during the critical
days of their menstrual cycle. In several workplaces, women have
organized Therapeutic Touch support teams so that they can help
each other during these trying times. They perform Therapeutic
Touch sessions for each other during lunch or morning or after-
noon breaks.

For fatigue, in addition to working on the areas mentioned
for the lethargic person, the following techniques are useful:

- Do Therapeutic Touch over the woman's neck muscles,
which act as repositories for the stress of physical exhaustion. Interface this energy work with gentle massage to
those muscles. Focusing on the penetration of the energy
field (or "poka-tru") over the nuchal (neck) muscles serves
to deeply relax them so that you may not have to spend a
great amount of time on the massage itself. As you do the
massage, consciously direct the energy of blue from your
hand chakras to and through the healee's musculature to
help release the stressed muscles.

- Also stimulate the healee's energy field by unruffling and supporting the energy flows to and through her foot chakras.

- There are several shiatsu or acupressure techniques that can be coupled with Therapeutic Touch. Used on the liver meridian, these techniques are particularly helpful for fatigue.

Depression is frequently reflected in a woman's posture—in the way she holds herself and the way she walks. In general, it involves lowered physical functioning and a despondent emotional response. Moreover, depression is contagious; when in the presence of a depressed person, you yourself may inadvertently reflect the depression without sufficient cause of your own to warrant such a state of dejection. Depression can be one of the spinoffs of protracted fatigue, particularly if the healee can see no way to get off the treadmill of certain work or life situations about which she is no longer enthusiastic. The following practices can assist the depressed person:

- There are many avenues of psychotherapeutic help that can support and nurture the healee's self-image and self-esteem. Counseling can offer many alternative choices in problem-solving.

- Rhythmic physical exercises such as aerobics and dancing, and rhythmic practices that raise the consciousness such as yoga, are very useful adjuncts to Therapeutic Touch for working with depression.

- In addition to the work mentioned previously for raising the healee's energy level, also work over the heart chakra for a depressed woman. To this interaction, bring a sense of deep caring; however, be very careful not to cloak it in a lather of sentimentality. The depressed woman has to be supported and encouraged to come to grips personally with the internal problems that set the stage for the depression. Otherwise, insight may elude her. Nevertheless, let her know that she is not alone.

- When doing unruffling to a depressed woman, do it for a few moments at a moderately brisk rate with the intention of facilitating the release of turgidity in the energy field and repatterning the energy flow.

The depressive state in PMS is usually transitory and has as much to do with hormonal imbalance as it does with psychic residue of the menarche experience. If symptoms of depression persist for a few weeks or more, the healee should seek the advice of a competent psychotherapist.

Depression can affect a woman in intangible and unexpected ways. The effect may at first be unobtrusive: a loss in appetite, or unusual overeating that may pass unnoticed. However, the psychological effect runs deeply. A breakdown in the sleep cycle and increasing but unexplainable irritability, fearfulness, or anxiety may occur. Frequently, these are accompanied by vague physical pains, unprovoked crying spells, and an inability to concentrate or remember. Moreover, this sorry state can be overlaid with an attitude of indifference and a loss of interest or pleasure in the daily activities of life. As the woman withdraws and loses confidence in her ability to handle life situations, the loss of self-esteem has insidious psychological consequences.

It can be very tiring to be around depressed people. They are known as "sappers" because they sap other people's vital energies. Some greedy ones are even "slurpers." They are usually low in energy and high in anxiety, so you have to be judicious in the way you conduct your healing interactions with such persons. Out of compassion, you must surely help those in need, but it is important that you exercise clear judgment about your own inner resources and ability to be therapeutic to others. Otherwise, you may become overwhelmed and possibly nontherapeutic.

To be therapeutic and also set limits with a depressed person, first be still and quietly center your consciousness. Then, when you are calm and able to feel unattached to the results of the healing interaction—that is, you do not have a personal investment in the outcome—send out a positive feeling such as affection to the needy healee, but at the same time set limits on the degree of your involvement. This willing, volitional act of setting limits neutralizes the draining effect of the sapper, it is said.

As noted several times, the emotional waters of the Therapeutic Touch interaction run deeply. Therefore, it is important to be discriminating in how you use your personal energies during the healing interaction. Emotional burnout is a rare complaint of persons who practice Therapeutic Touch; most practitioners feel a heightened sense of well-being from helping others in need. However, it is wise to be aware that there are extremes in the ways people choose to modify their energy fields and that not all modifications are in your best interest.

There are people of charisma and altruism who can stimulate your psyche and uplift your mood—the good teachers and good models. However, there are also those whose personal energy complexes are so devitalized that, as an act of survival, they reach out to other life-giving sources such as yourself that are offered to them. Under the best of conditions, you can set limits on your personal involvements with the sappers and slurpers of the world and on the duration of their Therapeutic Touch sessions.

When you yourself are tired or low in energy, you are most vulnerable to aggressive sappers or slurpers. These depressed people may not even realize what they are doing to others. If you feel that dealing with a healee's issue is too much for you, refer her to other therapeutic modalities that can serve her energy needs in a healthful manner and also be synergistic with your practice. From time to time, consult with the practitioners of these other modalities about the progress of the healee so that she has the benefit of many minds working on her problem.

To become aware of the wide spectrum of human energy levels, make it a practice to be alert to people's energy states as you walk through lobbies, down streets, or along shopping malls, and as you stand in lines at supermarkets or wait for traffic lights to change. Write your impressions of people's actions and behaviors in your journal.

When you have opportunities to do Therapeutic Touch assessments on energy-needy persons, be alert to the information that your hand chakras pick up about the nuances of their energy-flow dynamics, but be equally aware of your own reactions to the encounters, particularly the responses of your autonomic nervous system and your solar plexus chakra. Note your observations in your journal, and when you reread your notes, determine how you can make your future healing interactions with such persons both therapeutic for them and satisfying for yourself.

Water Retention, Abdominal Bloating, and Breast Engorgement

In PMS, water retention is related to fluid and electrolyte imbalance. It makes itself known by the presence of edematous (swollen) tissue, particularly around the woman's lower legs and ankles. However, the condition is often generalized so that not only the woman's shoes but the rest of her clothes feel tight and uncomfortable. Abdominal bloating is one manifestation of water retention. As a Therapeutic Touch practitioner, you can assist these conditions in the following way:

- Before the Therapeutic Touch session begins, take the healee's radial (wrist) pulse and blood pressure. You can also measure the circumference of the areas that are edematous. Repeat these measurements at the end of the session and keep them for your records.

- Although the liver looks like an undistinguished blob of red tissue, it is an exceedingly complex organ with more than forty functions, one of which is fluid and electrolyte balance. Therefore, begin the treatment by working over the liver and kidney-adrenal areas of the solar-plexus chakra complex. Modulate the energy over the liver by visualizing an emerald-green color. For kidney-adrenal energy modulation, a yellow-gold energy level is most useful.

- Briskly unruffle in an *upward* direction to clear the healee's energy field, stimulate it, and help it to repattern. In the case of dependent edema, intermittently concentrate your work on the legs and feet. Also support the foot chakras in the excretion of waste energies. To do this, have the healee's feet comfortably elevated so that gravity can aid the effort.

- From time to time, reassess the healee's energy field, particularly over her heart and solar-plexus chakra complexes to get a sense of the extent and quality of the rebalancing that has taken place.

- After the Therapeutic Touch session, when it is time for the healee to rest or nap, have her lie so that her legs are comfortably elevated but below the level of the heart.

- Also help the healee analyze her diet to pinpoint water-retaining foods or habits. Or, upon her request, refer her to a knowledgeable nutritionist.

Breast engorgement during PMS makes a woman's breasts tender to the touch or uncomfortable in restricting garments. If the woman feels up to it, cold compresses or an ice bag for short periods of time may prove helpful in relieving congestion in the breasts.

To further alleviate the discomfort of breast engorgement, use Therapeutic Touch techniques as follows:

- Place your hand chakras in the energy field overlying the breasts and gently unruffle the energy field in an attempt to disperse the congested energy flow.

- If the breasts continue to be painful, modulate the energy over them by visualizing the color blue and sending that wavelength of energy to the energy field overlying the painful area.

- It may be useful to have the healee do an imagery exercise that will promote the healing process. This imagery exercise could also be "homework" for the healee to do at a later time. As with all imagery practices it is important that the imagery chosen be relevant to the healee.

Persons Who Are HIV+

It is difficult to remember that until quite recently we were ignorant of the Human Immunodeficiency Virus (the AIDS virus) and the human misery it leaves in its wake as its pathological consequences rage throughout the world's population. A personal illustration of this stands out in my mind. In 1988, I was teaching a graduate research class how to do data retrieval in a computer lab. I thought it would be timely to call for a printout of the current literature on AIDS, which was very much on everyone's mind. Significant studies had begun to be reported in the mid-eighties, so we punched in a request for a 1985 bibliography on AIDS. The computer responded with an alacrity that drew exclamations of delight from the students, while I watched proudly as my shiny toy made short work of our requested search and promptly printed out several neat, clean pages of bibliography. However, my pride turned to chagrin when we collected the fan of printed papers and found that the computer search of 1985 literature on AIDS had resulted only in a list of studies on "hearing aids"! A year later, in 1986, the term AIDS was a household word.

Current theory holds that the HIV is a retrovirus, which means that it is capable of reversing the apparent normal flow of genetic information. One might say that AIDS is the final statement of a progressive immune disorder that has been silent for years. It is thought that in some as yet poorly understood manner, an important white blood cell, the macrophage, which is part of the immune system, may itself serve as a reservoir for the retrovirus.

AIDS has become pandemic. There is hardly a country in the world whose borders it has not penetrated. As an indication of the fear its spread has aroused, the United Nations recently reported that most of the merchants had fled from several towns in Africa (such as Kyotera in Uganda) and that most of these towns' children are now orphans. Stories from other parts of the world are equally pitiful, and scientific progress toward finding a "magic bullet" cure seems to be torturously slow.

It has become apparent that this is an exceedingly complex disease that calls for a multifaceted approach to healing. At this time, most treatments for AIDS are palliative and directed toward improvement of the quality of life, which itself is a noble undertaking.

To date, Therapeutic Touch has only been able to deal with the secondary, opportunistic infections that plague persons who are HIV+, and not all efforts at using Therapeutic Touch have been successful. However, over the past five years, many practitioners have worked with persons who are HIV+ as well as with their families, buddies, and friends to learn how Therapeutic Touch can be used most effectively on the effects of this plague. Most of the experiences have been with HIV+ adults, and almost all of these adults have been men.

Practitioners have also worked in hospitals with children of HIV+ mothers who were drug abusers. In New York City, which has one of the largest concentrations of HIV+ persons in the United States, it is estimated at this time that approximately one in seventy children has been exposed to the retrovirus. A growing number of these children whose mothers have died have been left at the hospitals to live out their short lives.

In an unexpected psychosocial happening, since 1989 an unusually large number of these children have been brought up by their grandparents, perhaps as surrogates for their own children, who are now dead. Or, the children have been adopted by buddies whose companions have died of the retrovirus infection. It is especially satisfying to report—as one act in an otherwise dispirited situation—that many of these people have learned to do Therapeutic Touch to the stricken children, and I am delighted to count them among Krieger's Krazies.

The number of symptoms with which Therapeutic Touch practitioners have been able to work successfully is painfully small. However, the results of the work are summarized below. It should be kept in mind that persons with AIDS have an immensely overworked immune system. They are greatly fatigued and are not able to absorb a large amount of prana, the vital life-force energy. Because of this, it is important to do Therapeutic Touch in frequent, short sessions with these persons.

As a healer working with persons with AIDS, it is also important that you have a strong psychological support system of your own, for you are working with an illness that is the tragedy of our times. It is also requisite that you have a deeply rooted personal philosophy of life and death.

Elevated Temperature

Compresses of cool, diluted alcohol or light cologne are comforting and helpful in reducing elevated temperature. Also use simple measures such as insuring adequate fluid intake along with the following:

- Moderately unruffle the healee's energy field. This technique dissipates the congestion and keeps the energy flowing freely.

- Modulate the healee's energy field with your hand chakras using blue energy.

- Use cotton pads charged with blue energy as described in Experiential Exercise 7 to bring down elevated temperatures. Place the charged cotton pads over the major pulses of the healee's body, much as you would place cool compresses.

Nausea and Vomiting

The Therapeutic Touch practitioner can help modify the conditions of nausea and vomiting as follows:

- Lightly place the palm of one hand on the healee's forehead and the other at the nape of the neck to inhibit retching.

- While helping the healee to be comfortable, stabilize the solar-plexus chakra complex, and modulate the energy field with blue energy.

- Gently unruffle the energy field as the seizures lessen, and facilitate the energy flow to and through the foot chakras.

- Intermittently calm and support the heart chakra.

- As the spasms cease, help the healee into a comfortable position, cover with a light blanket, and let him or her rest or nap.

All of the above Therapeutic Touch interactions are, of course, done in the healee's energy field.

Diarrhea

The fluid and electrolyte imbalance is frequently severe with diarrhea, and the convulsive gastrointestinal spasms are exhausting. Here are several things you can do for the healee:

- Stabilize the area of the solar plexus chakra complex and modulate the healee's energy field with blue energy.

- Modulate the energies over the liver and the spleen chakra with blue energy as well to help lessen the spasms.

- Take advantage of the resultant relaxation response to encourage the healee to rest and, if possible, to sleep. Because of the healee's weakened state, stay nearby to help should a contingency arise.

Headache

Therapeutic Touch works best with tension headaches caused by stress and with headaches that are in response to environmental conditions, such as the lowered barometric pressure that often precedes a thunderstorm. Headaches in a person who is HIV+

may be due to the process of the viral infection itself, or they may be nonspecific. Nevertheless, it is useful to bolster symptomatic control using the following techniques:

- Begin by lightly unruffling the energy field over the head, eyes, neck, and shoulders, using short, rapid, gentle movements of your hands.

- It is very comforting to stand behind the healee and then quietly and very lightly rest your hand chakras over the healee's eye sockets for a minute or two; this drains off some of the energy congestion.

- Coupling light massage, shiatsu, or acupressure with Therapeutic Touch modulation in the blue energy range to the muscles in the back of the neck and shoulders helps relieve congested energy flows.

- If the headache has been very painful or if it has continued over a long period of time, the stress may be considerable, even causing nausea; therefore, also stabilize the solar plexus chakra complex, using energies in the blue range.

- As the condition clears, modulate the healee's energy field in the blue energy range, using moderate, rhythmic movements.

- The release from pain, coupled with a relaxation response, may give the healee an opportunity to rest quietly or to sleep, the most potent regenerator of all.

Chemotherapy and Radiation Sickness

Chemotherapy and radiation therapy are heroic measures that are used only during critical stages of illness. It is expected that they have severe side effects. Because of this, I prefer to work preventively. I begin Therapeutic Touch sessions about a week before the healee is scheduled to begin chemotherapy or radiation therapy, directing my efforts toward stress reduction, psychosomatic stabilization, and any contingencies that may arise. As when I work with people who have carcinoma or sarcoma, either I avoid directing energies to the sites of the lesions or, if the occasion demands, I do Therapeutic Touch as follows, though very gently and sensitively and only for short periods at a time:

- To counteract the fear and anxiety, stabilize the solar plexus and heart chakra complexes with the energy of clear light.

- Place your hand chakras over the healee's breastbone (which overlies the thymus) and direct supporting energy flows to the healee's immune system.

- Work with the axis of the spleen chakra and liver, using a yellow-gold energy range over the spleen and an emerald green energy over the liver. Besides simply directing energy to them, attempt to integrate and balance their energy flows.

- In addition, direct yellow-gold energy to help strengthen and stabilize the solar plexus chakra complex, working particularly in the area of the kidney-adrenals.

- Together with the healee, work out imagery and meditative exercises as homework, and devise a schedule of daily fluid intake to assure that the healee is adequately hydrated before the chemotherapy or radiation therapy begins.

- If you have not done so previously, teach basic Therapeutic Touch skills to those relatives, buddies, or friends who want to help, and set up practice sessions for them.

- Continue Therapeutic Touch sessions throughout the chemotherapy or radiation therapy schedule. Your goal is to help the healee maintain equilibrium and to use Therapeutic Touch symptomatically.

Hospice

In my personal worldview, I perceive death as a natural and expected occurrence in the life continuum, with the light of consciousness providing connectivity. Therefore, I consider that even though a healee dies, the experiences that occur while the healee is living can provide a time of healing for both the healee and those who are of significance to him or her. For this reason, and if circumstances permit, I try to bring family members and friends into the Therapeutic Touch experience. Either I do Therapeutic Touch to them as a mode of stress reduction or, at their request or if they demonstrate an interest, I teach Therapeutic Touch skills to them so they can experience this unique intimacy with the healee.

There is thought to be a significant relationship between the *anahata* (heart) chakra and physical touch. Because of this, the following practice has developed among persons who work in hospice or elsewhere with people who are dying.

Sit quietly by the bedside as the time of transition approaches and, after centering, simultaneously touch the healee's hand chakra and the area of the heart chakra complex. Even if you are too overwhelmed by the circumstances to do anything else, simply use this time to send a sense of deep caring and love to the healee, and wish him or her well on the journey.

If you can do more to meet the healee's needs in these final moments, Dora Kunz suggests that you use Therapeutic Touch skills to convey to the healee a sense of peace and permission to go. She advises the direction of gentle, minimal energies alternating between the blue and yellow-gold ranges to the dying person, with the intention of conveying a sense of peace and the recognition that the healee is going into circumstances where there is no physical suffering.

Dora Kunz points out that your role as the healer in a time of sorrow is not to get involved in the turbulence of mixed emotions but to be emotionally stable and give to others the energy to bear their own feelings. In this way, you can be of service to the living as well as to those who are shifting to another state of consciousness.

Abdominal Operations and Caesarian Sections

Under the best of circumstances, start to work with a person about to undergo an abdominal operation or Caesarian section at least a few days before the operation. Some of this time can be spent discussing the forthcoming experience and helping the healee to complete plans for the hospitalization. For example, the healee can arrange for preregistration at the hospital so that the actual admission procedure occurs without incident. Also, suggest that the healee's diet include adequate fluid intake and that the healee rest during the preoperative days. Other details will probably be medically prescribed. In doing Therapeutic Touch at this time, your major objective is to elicit a relaxation response to reduce anxiety, promote rest, and give the healee a sense of comfort and well-being.

Once hospitalization has occurred, do Therapeutic Touch with the knowledge and permission of the healee's physician and the hospital administration, if that is required, and, of course, at the request of the healee. Also discuss your plans with the nurse administrator and work out a feasible schedule for your visits.

After the operation, Therapeutic Touch is helpful in restoring peristalsis. Therefore, it could be done by nurses knowledgeable of Therapeutic Touch while the healee is still in the recovery room. Therapeutic Touch also is helpful for nausea or vomiting, and for the reduction of postoperative anxiety and pain.

For various reasons, including poor circulation, it is possible for intravenous fluids to infiltrate the healee's surrounding tissues. As with edema, Therapeutic Touch can promote the reabsorption of fluids and reduce the swelling and discomfort. However, if the intravenous apparatus is in place and you are a layperson or not registered with the institution, the hospital administration may not allow your intervention. Under these conditions, offer to teach qualified staff persons to do the skill. Incidentally, Therapeutic Touch also helps the absorption and reduces the sting of intramuscular and subcutaneous injections.

Other Therapeutic Touch skills to use include unruffling and modulation with blue energy over the operative site (the solar plexus chakra) for pain or discomfort. Also, support the heart chakra complex for stress reduction, the liver-spleen chakra axis for elimination of toxic wastes, and the thymus for stimulating the healee's immune system and recuperative abilities. Your major objective at this time is to promote rest and the well-being of the healee; Therapeutic Touch effects a relaxation response that induces sleep or a nap, both of which promote healing.

As the discomfort recedes, work with yellow-gold energy over the spleen chakra and the kidney-adrenal area of the solar plexus chakra complex to promote pranic intake and absorption. Also work to facilitate the systemic energy flow to and through the foot chakras.

You can integrate into your Therapeutic Touch practice a number of other healing modalities:

- To help the healee relax and to fully ventilate and clear the lungs, teach the healee breathing exercises.

- After the healee has been in bed for a few continuous days, he or she will greatly appreciate a light massage of the back and feet. The aroma of the cedar or juniper oil used in the massage is very refreshing for someone who has been bedfast.

- Simple joint exercises assure adequate circulation. There are some very effective, easily assumed yoga positions that the healee can do in bed without strain to the abdominal muscles.[8]

- Neck tension can be relieved by integrating acupressure with Therapeutic Touch. Use acupoints on the scalp and neck (B10, GB20, TW16) and on the top of the shoulders (GB21). The acupressure can also be done by the healee.[9]

• As homework, incorporate imagery of the healee's choice that is synergistic with the healing process.

During the recuperative period, continue support with whatever Therapeutic Touch skills are appropriate and encourage the healee to do as much as is sensible in the interest of his or her well-being. Read Ryan's *The Fine Art of Recuperation*, which advocates that the healee make efforts toward independence; it is written in a most refreshing fashion.[10]

A Caesarian section is an abdominal operation. But it is also more, since it is done on a pregnant woman who has gone through several months of critical endocrinal and physiological changes and who is carrying within herself a new life. Caesarian sections are meant to be done in cases of difficult or dangerous childbirth. However, an air of convenience has entered the decision-making process with regard to childbirth, so that at this time one in four childbirths in large cities occur by Caesarian section, without regard to the criticality of the birthing condition.

In addition to working with the suggestions given for abdominal operations, preoperatively teach the husband, family member, or close friend a few basic and appropriate Therapeutic Touch skills.

• Postoperatively, do Therapeutic Touch to relieve engorged breasts and to promote milk flow.

• For cracked nipples, use the same skills you would for wound healing and reduction of pain.

• Teach the parents how to do Therapeutic Touch to their new baby, as well as to their other children.

How You Know

Specific methods for using Therapeutic Touch skills with dozens of symptoms have been discussed so far. However, unless you do the experiential exercises and practice your skills on living beings, these discussions are only intellectual exercises for you.

It is the human feedback you receive in the actual practice of these skills that is essential for a valid understanding of the Therapeutic Touch process.

Underlying these skills is the basic assumption that your charge as the healer is to rebalance the healee's energy field. Since you are concerned with the balancing of energies, are you doing the same thing with both of your hands? Experiential Exercise 12 has been designed to help you come to your own conclusions.

EXPERIENTIAL EXERCISE 12

Using the Hand Chakras to Rebalance the Healee's Energy Field

This experiential exercise can be done as a guided imagery to help you reexperience your last Therapeutic Touch interaction with a healee, or you can keep the steps in mind and make the decisions that are called for during your next Therapeutic Touch interaction with someone who is ill.

Do this exercise in a quiet place, when you can be assured that you will have twenty minutes of uninterrupted time to fully experience your recollections.

Equipment

Have a pen and paper pad nearby so that you can easily jot down your impressions.

Procedure

1. Sit in a comfortable position and quietly center your consciousness.

2. As you stay on center, go back in your memory to the last Therapeutic Touch interaction you had with a healee.

3. Be there in your mind's eye, standing next to the healee. Feel the presence of his or her energy field.

4. Clearly visualize your interacting human energy fields as

your hand chakras respond to field cues in your assessment of the healee's condition.

5. Now make a decision on how you can best help the healee and begin to rebalance his or her energy field.

6. As you rebalance, pay particular attention to how your hand chakras are functioning. What information are you receiving from them?

7. How are you using your dominant and nondominant hand chakras? Are their functions the same? Different?

8. Write down your impressions on the pad of paper as the answers are clarified for you.

9. If you are doing this exercise with other persons, discuss your findings.

Comments on Exercise 12

As you may now perceive, each of your hand chakras may be engaged in a different function and may perform differently from the other one during the rebalancing of the healee's energy field. A recent class of seventy Therapeutic Touch practitioners shared their perceptions of how they were using their nondominant hand chakras while their dominant hand chakras were actively directing or modulating energy flow. They said that the nondominant hand chakra

- provides the dominant hand chakra with a basis for comparison;
- is the "listener"—it checks and validates the effect of the dominant hand chakra's direction or modulation of energy flow;
- draws energy to the area, and distributes and balances the energy flow;

- sets up the parameters of a therapeutic energy field and maintains the field's focus;
- balances and supports the energy field;
- helps the healee's energy field ground or anchor the therapeutic energy flow.

Other Examples of Therapeutic Touch in Practice

The instances of Therapeutic Touch practice cited throughout this book represent just a few of the many ways that Therapeutic Touch is being used. Professional persons in the health field use Therapeutic Touch in hundreds of situations that cover a wide spectrum; some are unusual, others are quite funny. Following are a few examples that may be of interest to you:

- In one town, a Krieger's Krazy has a Therapeutic Touch practice set up in the locker room of a well-known football team. She does Therapeutic Touch on the sports injuries of the football players. In a neighboring town, another practitioner is doing research on the effects of Therapeutic Touch on E. coli (a microscopic organism) at the county sewage plant.

- In a modern, high-tech hospital of a city, Therapeutic Touch is a routine procedure done on premature babies in the neonatal intensive care unit. On a farm several miles beyond the city's limits, a farmer uses Therapeutic Touch in his hen house to increase the egg-laying efficiency of a flock of Rhode Island Reds.

- In another part of the country, a male nurse has set up an after-hours Therapeutic Touch practice in the back of a bar for injured alcoholics and others who would otherwise not seek out health care. During the day, a medical doctor who works in that state's prison teaches prisoners the basic skills of Therapeutic Touch.

A Few Suggestions

Here are a few suggestions that may be useful to you in your practice of Therapeutic Touch:

- Keep objective records of the various Therapeutic Touch skills you use, the various conditions under which they are used, and the results you have with them. At a later time, compare the skills you use to pick up cues during assessment or reassessment with the skills you use to rebalance energy. Note the similarities and differences you find in various patterns of energy flow, and try to clarify for yourself why you use certain rebalancing skills and how you use them under various circumstances. This analysis may seem tedious, but once you understand the repertoire of skills you put into use, your knowledgeable and discriminating use of Therapeutic Touch can become a powerful tool to help others in need.

- Compare notes with your friends or colleagues who also practice Therapeutic Touch. Develop a communications network among these people so that you can confer with each other by phone, electronic bulletin boards, and so on, and learn from each other's experiences.

- Translate your findings into inferences about the healing process, and discuss their implications with persons in other healing modalities who may have other perspectives.

- Consider under which conditions the techniques of other modalities might be usefully coupled with Therapeutic Touch skills to meet the needs of healees.

- Continually sharpen your sensitivity to those you can help; however, use your best judgment in opening yourself to new situations. By objectively reviewing your journal of Therapeutic Touch experiences once a month or so, it will become clear to you which habits of thought you can trust and under which conditions you act with clarity.

• Use notes on the contents of your dreams, spontaneous imageries, and meditations to understand your own motivations in wanting to be a healer and the effects they are having on your inner life.

Cautions and Precautions

• Hippocrates's admonition "Do no harm" has been passed down for twenty-five hundred years as excellent advice for anyone who would help or heal others. Harm most frequently occurs because of ignorance. Therefore, if you don't know what to do, refer the healee to someone who does. Or, if upon reassessment you pick up no further cues in the healee's energy field, do not just perseverate; assure yourself of the healee's comfort and safety, and stop the Therapeutic Touch interaction. Human energies are not well understood at this time, but we do know that indiscriminate and persistent interactions can overload the human system; a healee can overdose on human energies. A useful rule of thumb to keep in mind as you learn about Therapeutic Touch is to underdo rather than overdo. Invariably, you can come back at a later time and continue Therapeutic Touch if it is warranted.

• In a healing modality such as Therapeutic Touch, in which you yourself are the major conduit through which energies are being specifically directed or sensitively modulated for the well-being of another, it is of utmost importance that you have confidence in what you are doing. Confidence arises from certainty about what you are doing. Therefore, in the Therapeutic Touch rebalancing of energy flow, do only what you know from the assessment and the reassessment. The cues you pick up are direct communications from the healee's energy field and provide a thoughtful basis for knowledgeable intervention. You might also find it useful to have a videocamera in operation as you practice Therapeutic Touch so that you can observe yourself objectively at a later time and thus gain confidence. When you review the interaction, do not look only at what you are doing. Listen carefully to any dialogue between yourself and the healee. Notice the healee's body language and posture during the session. Ask yourself, What else could I have learned about the individual? How else could I have helped him or her?

- Never sweat. Energy flow is natural and occurs effortlessly. Don't push. Only in rare instances will you have to exert force of any kind. Your major purpose in doing Therapeutic Touch is to help the healee stimulate or modify energy flow and to reestablish rhythm to that flow. The direction and modulation of human energy flow originates in the mind and is empowered by the mind. It entails a facile, nonphysical employment of the therapeutic use of self. If you are in doubt about what to do, place your hand chakras in the energy field overlying the healee's kidney-adrenals, or place them in direct contact with that region of the healee's back (at approximately the level of the lowest ribs). Simply allow the energized flow to occur naturally between you. As noted previously, this simple technique for energy transfer has never been injurious to anyone, and most recipients feel an elevated energy level and experience a sense of well-being.

- Use Therapeutic Touch sensitively, gently, and for short periods with pregnant women, children, persons with head injuries or lesions, persons experiencing much trauma who may be in shock, persons in fragile health, and psychologically disabled persons (who usually like Therapeutic Touch very much but may become frightened by sudden movements).

- Nevertheless, never fail to try to help, even if the odds are against the situation. At least three persons who were catatonic (in three institutions that were widely separated), for whom attending psychiatrists held out little hope, responded in some significant manner to Therapeutic Touch. A woman who had been catatonic for eighteen years relaxed her spastic arms, which had been held in severe contractions all those years, and smiled. Although she did not speak, thereafter she was amenable to care, got into a wheelchair every morning, and seemed alert and genuinely more interested in daily activities. A nineteen-year-old boy came out of his catatonic state and asked for a glass of water and the name of the nurse who had done Therapeutic Touch to him. Very recently, another catatonic lady spoke for the first time in twenty years. Her first word was the nickname of the nurse who had been doing Therapeutic Touch with her the past several weeks.

• Use objective criteria: Did the Therapeutic Touch help? If the illness was healed, were there secondary effects? Did it translate into something else?

Legal Implications

Individual state laws vary, but in general laypersons are allowed to practice healing within their own families or if it is an essential expression of their religious beliefs. In the health professions, Therapeutic Touch is regarded as an extension of professional skills. Nevertheless, I suggest that each person examine the state practice act for their own profession to make sure there is no legal conflict with the practice of Therapeutic Touch. In most states, health practitioners come under the state medical practice act. Physicians, psychiatrists, and psychologists have independent practices. Professional nurses have an independent nurse practice act in the majority of states.

There is a provision in the federal laws for tax deductions for "unconventional practitioners." Commenting on the interpretation of these deductions, *Consumer Reports* states: "In short, a medical expense is any amount paid to make you healthy when you are sick, or to preserve your health when you have a specific chronic ailment.[11]

Chapter 6

A REVIEW

When performing Therapeutic Touch, you learn about the functional uses of the human energy field; however, to make this knowledge your own, you must be willing to use senses other than the five major ones. As mentioned previously, Therapeutic Touch entails a different kind of intelligence than is used in the conventional daily activities of living. It involves other ways of communicating within yourself and with others—ways that utilize poorly understood functions of the psyche. The point of entry for this healing system is the farther reaches of consciousness. This realm of the deep self is invoked by the irresistible upsurge of compassionate concern for the welfare of another. It is a concern of such depth of feeling that it impels you to exceed the usual grasp of things.

Under the best of conditions, the facets of consciousness that are fostered by the practice of Therapeutic Touch include validated personal knowledge, well-grounded mind-to-mind transmission of information between healer and healee (i.e., telepathy), and the skillful use of intuition and creative thought. Such possible acquisitions constitute a very heady set of abilities. So what is the source of the state of consciousness necessary to obtain these abilities?

The answer lies somewhere between the motivation to help or heal, whose roots are nurtured by a compassionate concern for those in need, and the persistent drive to shape yourself as a beneficent human support system geared toward this altruistic goal. This healing path involves hard work, but not of the sweaty variety. It takes a deep-seated commitment, willingness, and self-discipline to naturally awakening your latent abilities for the service of the good. However, I would like to emphasize the fact that this is a natural awakening, for it is my conviction that healing, as it occurs in Therapeutic Touch, is a natural potential that can be actualized by anyone under the appropriate circumstances. An even deeper grasp of the farther reaches of consciousness involved in the healing process may occur when you utilize the more advanced techniques of Therapeutic Touch.

The Context of Therapeutic Touch Practice

Without a doubt, the most unique proposition that has been presented in this book is that as humans we do not stop at our skins. In fact, a fount of important information characteristic of the authentic self lies waiting to be tapped in the dynamic circuitry of the energy field just beyond the skin. A functioning or healthy portion of this energy field can be used as a model of the healthy, integrated energetic processes of a healee. You as the healer can then perceive cues about the healee's energy imbalances by picking them up in contrast to this normal background. Through an analysis or assessment of these cues, you then can help rebalance the ill person's energy field by utilizing a series of cue-specific techniques.

In review, the process of Therapeutic Touch could be said to have four phases. The first phase, centering the consciousness, is a constant and is the ground state from which Therapeutic Touch proceeds. The other phases are in no way timebound, and they fade in and out as circumstances demand. The second phase is assessment, or searching the healee's energy field for cues indicative of imbalance. The third phase is rebalancing, or repatterning, the energy deficits, hyperactivity, blockages, or dysrhythmias. The fourth phase involves making an informed decision based on frequent reevaluations of the healee's energy field about when to discontinue or redirect the healing interaction. It is through this reassessment that you realize whether Therapeutic Touch has been of help and get a sense of the next steps to take for the healee's well-being.

The Centering Phase

Centering the consciousness establishes the basis for a continuum of awareness throughout the Therapeutic Touch process, the ultimate goal being to induce a ceaseless flow of consciousness from the deep reaches of the self. Centering is an experience in focusing within the self. It is a uniquely personal way of relating to the depths of yourself and then using the perspective gained as a touchstone or gauge of internal validity in the healer-healee interaction.

The Assessment Phase

In the assessment phase, you maintain this centered state of consciousness and use your own chakras (vortices of consciousness), primarily those in the energy field of the palms of your hands, to sense the healee's energy-field flow patterns. These energy patterns have several characteristics:

Flow. The flow of the energy may range from:

- slow to fast
- unimpeded to congested
- strong to weak
- tenuous to full
- quiet to tumultuous
- pulsating to pounding

Rhythm. The intrinsic rhythm of the energy may range from:

- cadent to arrhythmic
- regular to random
- harmonic to dissonant

Resonance. The energy can bring certain physical body systems such as the autonomic nervous system into sympathetic resonance with its flows and rhythms, for example, the "gut reaction" to the emotional energy of fear.

In your assessment of imbalance, you learn to differentiate amongst the various energy flows, rhythmicities, and effects on the physical, emotional, intellectual, and suprarational systems. As noted previously, there are six major indicators of imbalance that most people are capable of distinguishing:

- Temperature differentials of heat or cold
- Attraction or magnetic pull to an area
- Energy deficit or hyperactivity
- Congestion or blockage of energy flow
- Tingling or slight electric shocks
- Pulsations or unsynchronized rhythms

It is interesting to note that these imbalance indicators arise directly out of the human-energy-field interaction between healer and healee. For example, a healee's energy field may not be intrinsically "hot" or "tingly"; instead, this description arises out of your attempt as the healer to verbalize your experience during the assessment.

There are also Therapeutic Touch practitioners who learn how to use their intuitive abilities reliably, and others who learn over time how to become cognizant of information filtered through their chakra complexes. Yet other practitioners integrate a variety of abilities or practices into their use of Therapeutic Touch, often with very useful results. For instance, I was taught how to ascertain the twelve pulses of acupuncture using sensitive contact touch. When I want to fine-tune or cross-match the information I pick up from a healee's energy field during an assessment, I also find it useful to assess the energy field over these pulses. (I don't actually touch the skin.) In particular, I find the large intestine pulse to be very helpful.

One thing I do not do, or do only with great care, is accept the healees' own diagnoses of their own problems. I would suggest that you also use caution in doing so. Frequently, healees' problems fill them with anxiety that may cloud or bias their descriptions or conclusions, and blind acceptance may send you off in the wrong direction. For instance, it is not always the case that problems lie where healees feel pain. In referred pain, healees may, for example, feel pain shooting down their left arms when in fact their problems are cardiac in origin; this occurs with angina pectoris. Or they may feel pain below their shoulder blades when their actual problems are with their gall bladder.

Over the years, I have found that the most reliable method for ascertaining the problem is to "listen" to my hand chakras and to focus on interpreting the messages I receive clearly. Nevertheless, if there is a matter of pain, I do listen very carefully to the healee post-treatment to find out whether what I was doing to relieve the pain was in fact helpful. If it was not, I either do something else or I refer the healee to someone who can help.

There are many possible reasons for the existence of different symptoms. Therefore, I recommend that, in conjunction with learning Therapeutic Touch, you study an up-to-date edition of a reliable medical source book. The *American Medical Association Family Medical Guide* is very good, particularly the section containing the self-diagnosis symptom charts.[1] These charts are a series of decision-tree diagrams that offer clear explanations about a wide variety of symptom groups. This book also outlines simple methods for alleviating some symptoms and, most importantly, outlines specific indications of possible emergency situations. As an example, the following are all possible causes for the symptom of chest pain:

- heart attack
- blood clot in the lungs
- bronchitis
- heartburn

- hiatus hernia
- chest injury
- pulled muscle
- fractured rib
- nerve infection, such as shingles
- pneumonia or pneumothorax (a collection of air or gas in the pleural cavity), if the chest pain is coupled with elevated temperature

The Rebalancing Phase

Once an assessment of the healee's energy field is determined, your objective then shifts to an attempt to rebalance the healee's energy field. As a general guide, it is important to keep the principle of opposites in mind. If the healee's energy flows seem closed or congested, attempt to stimulate or open them. If the flows are chaotic, attempt to calm them. If there is tension, release the stress.

Movement. In the rebalancing phase of the Therapeutic Touch process, you can use movement in several ways. In general, the direction of your hand-chakra movements should be from the crown of the healee's head toward the feet, for reasons discussed in earlier chapters. However, should your assessment indicate the need, the direction of movement in certain areas can be varied. Bringing your hand chakras down through the healee's energy field is usually relaxing, whereas moving them upward is stimulating. In either action, the palms of your hands should face the direction of movement, and your fingers should be relaxed but held next to one another. The quality of the movements themselves should express the effect you are trying for, so they can be brisk, moderate, or gentle as the occasion demands. As previously discussed, it is your own attention or focus of mind as the healer that directs or modulates the energy flow and makes it more coherent and organized. Therefore, the process is greatly enhanced by visualization, which focuses and coordinates the effort and brings to it a measure of control. Focus can also be sharpened with the breath, by directing the energy flow as you exhale.

Another movement of the hands you can call upon is unruffling. Unruffling movements are directed at moving energy from the inner, more central area of the healee's energy field outward, toward its periphery. Unruffling serves many purposes, including decongesting an area of the energy field that appears to be blocked, changing an energy pattern, or cooling an elevated body temperature or area of inflammation.

Body movement by the healee can also be useful in Therapeutic Touch practice. For example, when working with a healee who has joint problems, I find it very useful to have the healee slowly rotate the affected extremity while I assess the energy field over the joint. Very often I feel a decided change in the energy flow over a particular part of the joint during the rotation. This gives me a clearer idea of the healee's problem and indicates where I should direct my efforts during Therapeutic Touch.

Another type of movement that has proven itself helpful during Therapeutic Touch was developed by Dora Kunz. It is useful for problems with locomotion, such as those that occur following the fracture of a leg, and involves directing the energy flow along the long bones of the legs, behind the knees, and then out through the feet chakras (in the energy field over the arches of the feet). (See figure 3.) After the healee has had this Therapeutic Touch, he or she is properly supported (either by apparatus or by other persons) and asked to walk a short distance. This exercise naturally and functionally patterns the energy flow and accelerates the healing process. A similar ploy can be used with musculoskeletal problems of the upper extremities; that is, they can be put through a functional range of motion to facilitate normal energy flow following a Therapeutic Touch session.

I find hydrotherapy to be a useful adjunct with these practices, and I do Therapeutic Touch while the healees, and sometimes myself, are in the moving waters. My place of choice to do this is in natural, living waters such as hot springs, active rivers or streams, or protected coves along the seacoast where the essential nature of the waters themselves may suggest to the hand chakras the multiple patterns of natural energy flow.

Modulating Energy Flow. Modulating human energies is somewhat different from directing them. Modulating involves redistributing the healee's energies (rather than just pumping them in or out) or toning the quality or intensity of hyper- or hypoactive energy states. The visualization of specific colors and the empathic reflection within yourself of the distinctive energy states of these colors form the background of this skill.

By empathizing or identifying with a particular color, you reflect the energy state of that color in your body tone and then use this energy state to modulate or modify the healee's energy level. Symbols, music, and emotions can also be used to effect a modulation of energy in the healee. Below are listed several terms that Therapeutic Touch practitioners have used to describe the energy states they associate with specific colors.

COLOR	ENERGY STATE DESCRIPTIONS
blue	cool, quiet, composed, "waveless," peaceful, orderly, coherent, tranquil, a state of grace
yellow	vitalizing, highly mobile, invigorating, "pure energy," stimulating, active, quickening
green	equilibrium, dynamic stability, organized, balance
pink	affection, tenderness, love, sympathy, gentleness, enfoldment
violet	blessing, exalted, devotion, aspiring, dedication
clear light	clarity, accessible, translucence, permeable, unobstructed, unconditional

Rhythm. As noted previously, the prevalent energy used in the practice of Therapeutic Touch is prana. From the Indian perspective, prana is concerned with the organization that underlies the life process. Prana is actually an aspect of *vayu*, from which the rhythms in nature (i.e., cyclic phenomena) are derived. It is not surprising, therefore, that rhythm is one of the major avenues by which energy patterns are appreciated and understood during Therapeutic Touch. In this context, it is also interesting that problems related to rhythms are all strongly amenable to Therapeutic Touch intervention. This includes problems of the major rhythmic organs of the body such as the heart, the respiratory organs, the gastrointestinal tract, and the genitourinary system.

It also includes functional problems that are controlled by cyclic phenomena such as menses and pregnancy, and repetitive emotional problems such as manic depression.

With practice, rhythms in the human energy field are readily perceptible, particularly grossly abnormal rhythms. When you do Therapeutic Touch assessments on persons whose natural rhythms are being mechanically controlled, your overwhelming impression is of the dysrhythmias in their energy fields. This includes persons experiencing forced rhythmic breathing in respirators, or persons with severe renal problems using kidney dialysis machines that robotically filter their fluids and electrolytes in nonhuman rhythms.

Moreover, when patients are given high doses of antibiotics or psychotropics, or when they undergo chemotherapy, their energy flows feel out of sync and their timing out of phase. Such conditions need considerable experience to understand and work with. However, a great deal of good can be done for these people even with basic Therapeutic Touch techniques that invoke a simple relaxation response. It is remarkable how this response gives the body a momentary respite, during which it may regroup its forces and exercise its own intelligence in the effort to rebalance itself.

Chakras

Rhythm irregularity may be perceived during the Therapeutic Touch assessment in the chakras of the healee's energy field.

Chakras, as noted previously, are nonphysical vortices in the matrix of the human energy field that transform universal life-support energies into human energy systems. The locations and functions of the major chakras are closely related to the endocrine system and the autonomic nervous system. They are concerned with the input and output of the vital energies, which are in a state of constant flux.[2]

The dynamic of metabolism is a fundamental characteristic of all living beings and is essential for the regeneration of tissues— or healing—to take place. The finely tuned relationship between the chakras and the endocrine system offers you as the healer access to those energies called emotions and, thereby, to psychosomatic illnesses. The importance of the chakra complexes is made apparent by the fact that in excess of 70 percent of human illnesses in our stress-laden world are considered to be psychosomatic in origin.

However, the details of chakra functioning are not clearly apparent during the Therapeutic Touch assessment. You must rely on perceptible cues for hints of chakra malfunctioning, and it is important to validate such cues.

The most useful way I have found to understand the effect of chakras on awareness, behavior, attitude, and mood is to become aware of their functioning in myself. This strategy is utterly pragmatic, and I approach it as I would a game.

First, I recognize that the information about the chakras that has come from the East has been experientially validated over the past four thousand years. This to me is a rational basis upon which to proceed.

I then choose a chakra function that is common, simple, and agreed upon, such as the love function of the heart chakra. At a time when I will not be disturbed and am free to turn my full attention to the experience, I quietly center my consciousness. Then, in the case of experiencing the love function, and while maintaining a state of nonstressful but alert awareness, I clearly visualize someone whom I love and allow myself to feel love toward that person. I note clearly on every level of consciousness of which I am aware what is happening within myself as I deepen the experience of love.

When I do this exercise, I generally find that my respirations are calm and even and my muscles relaxed. I feel a general sense of comfort and well-being. Usually I like the way I feel—I may even find myself smiling—and, in reflection, my manner of relating to others is softened and more generous.

As I continue my exploration of this love facet of my consciousness, I begin understanding what is happening at deeper levels of my heart chakra. I ask myself, If I send loving thoughts to my true love, will that person respond in kind? The answer I receive is very frequently, yes. If I send loving thoughts to another, will that person open up to me? Very frequently, yes. If I send loving thoughts to a frightened child, will the child accept me? Very frequently, yes, and sometimes in unexpected and precious ways.

In a similar way, I go on to explore the other chakras. Over time, I get an added understanding of the fear that convulses the solar plexus chakra, the grief that grips the throat chakra, and so on. The psychosomatic outworkings of these stressed states then become clearer to me, and I begin to create therapeutic strategies for helping persons whose health is affected by these problems. The added knowledge that I gain from these experiences increases my repertoire of skills as this continuing quest makes me more sensitive to cues in the healee's energy fields. All that I learn I incorporate into my approach with Therapeutic Touch.

In the rebalancing phase of Therapeutic Touch, I place my hand chakras over the appropriate chakra in the healee's energy field. I then bring my own chakras into use by deeply centering and calling forth within myself the mind-set that incorporates the energetic qualities of the appropriate chakras. I use this spectrum of energies in the healer-healee interaction, much as I use the visualization of colors or rhythms for direction or modulation. In a short while, I look for a characteristic response in the healee's energy field that is a sympathetic resonance or reverberation of the healee's chakra complex with my own hand chakras. As with the other Therapeutic Touch practices, moderation and a knowledgeable basis for judgment are imperative. Therefore, I continue this interaction only for a short period of time, approximately two to three minutes. After this time, I do a reevaluation of the healee's energy field to determine my next course of action. The major areas to which I look for responses are the healee's endocrine system, autonomic nervous system, and emotions.

Conjoint Practices

Therapeutic Touch can be coupled with other healing modalities that may be helpful to the healee's well-being. Several of the following combinations have produced notable results:

- Therapeutic Touch interfaces very well with both physiotherapy and massage in cases of tension headache, other stress-related problems, low back pain, circulatory problems, and constipation. Physiotherapy is particularly helpful for the mobilization of joints and musculoskeletal dysfunctions.

- The combination of Therapeutic Touch and shiatsu or acupressure is very helpful in cases of sinusitis, digestive problems, fibrositis, muscular cramps, insomnia, and menstrual or menopausal problems.

- The combination of Therapeutic Touch and yoga works well for cases of bronchitis, asthma, varicose veins, high and low blood pressure, extreme fatigue, and anxiety reaction.

- Therapeutic Touch works very well with "homework" exercises in imagery in some hysterias, depression, panic syndrome, and during labor and delivery.

Putting into practice what you have learned will help you to ground the material and make it your own. Following is an exercise in guided imagery. It has been designed to help reinforce what you have learned about the practice of Therapeutic Touch. Either have someone read the material to you while you follow the instructions, or read the material yourself into a tape recorder and then play it back while you follow the instructions. The reading should be done slowly enough for you to experience the imagery.

EXPERIENTIAL EXERCISE 13

The Nature of Therapeutic Touch

Materials

Paper and pen should be nearby so that you can quickly make notes at each stage of the exercise. Make the notes brief and fill in details later so that you don't interrupt your flow of imagery.

Procedure

1. Go back in your mind's eye to a recent instance in which you used Therapeutic Touch. See yourself approaching the healee. What do you notice about him or her?

2. Stand beside the healee and take a moment to center your consciousness.

3. Do an assessment on the healee. How are you envisioning the healee's energy field? From where within yourself are you sensing his or her energies?

4. How will you treat the healee? How did you arrive at your decision? What will you do first? How would you explain what you are doing as you rebalance the energies?

5. How do you know that what you are doing is working? How do you think the healee has responded?

6. What do you think will happen as a result of this treatment?

7. What would you consider doing with this healee at the next Therapeutic Touch session? Why?

8. Take a deep breath, slowly open your eyes, and complete your journal.

Comments on Exercise 13

You can use this exercise at any time to objectively evaluate your progress.

The Miracle of Therapeutic Touch

Some months ago a friend, the renowned philosopher Renee Weber, Ph.D.,[3] pointed out to me that the teaching of Therapeutic Touch has marked the first time in Western history that healing has been routinely included in the formal curriculums of colleges and universities. I have been very grateful for the challenge of intellectual rigor that has been so much a part of the development of Therapeutic Touch as a contemporary interpretation of ancient healing practices. However, the techniques of Therapeutic Touch do not require exhaustive intellectual study; they are not difficult. What is essential to the process is what you, the healer, do with yourself. Healing is a humanization of energy, and Therapeutic Touch is a natural human potential. It is not a miracle cure. The miracle is that Therapeutic Touch can be done by everyone—including you.

COUNTRIES WHERE THERAPEUTIC TOUCH HAS BEEN TAUGHT

1972-1992

Afghanistan
Argentina
Australia
Austria
Belgium
Bolivia
Cambodia
Canada
Columbia
Czechoslovakia
Denmark
Dominican Republic
Egypt
England
Ethiopia
Finland
France
Georgia
Germany
Greece
Greenland
Guam
Holland

Hong Kong
Hungary
India
Mongolia
Iran
Ireland
Israel
Italy
Jamaica
Japan
Jordan
Kenya
Lebanon
Liberia
Luxembourg
Malaysia
Mauritius
Mexico
Nepal
New Guinea
New Zealand
Nigeria
Pakistan

People's Republic of China
Philippines
Poland
Russia
Scotland
Singapore
South Korea
Spain
Sri Lanka
Sweden
Switzerland
Taiwan
Tanzania
Thailand
Ukraine
Republic of South Africa
United States
Uruguay
Wales
Zaire
Zambia
Zimbabwe

SELF-EVALUATION OF THERAPEUTIC TOUCH SCALE

The Self-Evaluation of Therapeutic Touch Scale (SETTS) was developed in 1983 by Dolores Krieger and Patricia Winstead-Fry, Ph.D., R.N., at New York University as a measuring tool to distinguish persons who are experienced in the practice of Therapeutic Touch from those who are inexperienced. Although valid research findings are relevant only within a particular context, SETTS is reproduced below as an informal gauge of your interior or subjective experience with Therapeutic Touch techniques. As you proceed with this study of your own increasing expertise, SETTS will help clarify for you the nature of the act of centering, which is so central to the Therapeutic Touch process and to the powers of mindfulness that it fosters.

Instructions

The following items reflect experiences that Therapeutic Touch practitioners have had while performing Therapeutic Touch on healees. For each of the items, mark the frequency with which the experience occurs to you while you are engaged in the process of Therapeutic Touch, using the following scale:

0—not at all

1—once in a while

2—frequently

3—almost always

4—all the time

Therapeutic Touch Practitioner
Experience Survey

RATING	YOUR EXPERIENCE OF THERAPEUTIC TOUCH
☐	1. My heart and respiration rates feel slower.
☐	2. My breathing becomes slower and deeper.
☐	3. I feel sensations of heat and cold in my hands.
☐	4. I feel tingling sensations in my hands.
☐	5. I feel pressure in my hands.
☐	6. I feel electric shock sensations in my hands.
☐	7. I feel energy pulsations in my hands.
☐	8. I have the feeling that my hands are being spontaneously drawn to a particular area in the healee's field.
☐	9. I feel heat coming from my hands.
☐	10. I seem to be able to maintain uncomfortable postures much longer than usual.
☐	11. I seem to stand or kneel straighter than usual.
☐	12. My body movements become subtle, soft, and flowing.
☐	13. I become very sensitive to how I move my body and whether I am in an awkward or stressful position.
☐	14. My movements feel slow, steady, smooth, and alert.
☐	15. I feel energy moving through me and out of my hands.
☐	16. Energy flows more freely in my body.

☐ 17. I get a sense of stillness and balance in my body, mind, and emotions.

☐ 18. My body feels in harmony and seems to be an instrument through which energy flows.

☐ 19. My body feels quiet, calm, and relaxed.

☐ 20. I feel energy flowing rhythmically and evenly within my body.

☐ 21. I feel physically balanced, lined up, or integrated.

☐ 22. I feel as though all the parts of my body are working in unison.

☐ 23. I have a sense of physical and psychological attunement.

☐ 24. All my senses are heightened and sharpened.

☐ 25. I feel very close to the person I am healing.

☐ 26. I feel impersonal love for the healee, regardless of whether I liked the person before or not.

☐ 27. I feel loving and accepting toward myself and the healee.

☐ 28. I am more aware of my own emotions.

☐ 29. My own emotions seem to be set aside during the healing process.

☐ 30. I feel a sense of calmness, peace, and inner strength.

☐ 31. I feel detached and purposeful.

☐ 32. I feel an increase in sensitivity.

☐ 33. I feel an increase in empathy.

☐ 34. I feel an increase in compassion.

☐ 35. Emotions of love and peace feel like waves of energy going through me to the healee.

☐ 36. I am aware of the emotions of the healee as different qualities of energy.

☐ 37. I feel joy.

☐ 38. I trust that I have understanding at a level other than my conscious experience.

☐ 39. I have a sense of the Therapeutic Touch process being a totally integrated, flowing interaction.

☐ 40. I feel expansiveness.

☐ 41. I see spontaneous mental images that let me know what is going on in the healee.

☐ 42. I am more aware of the healee and less aware of activity going on in the surrounding environment.

☐ 43. When I focus attention on my hands and my feelings, the external environment seems to recede.

☐ 44. When I am focusing on the Therapeutic Touch process, my mind seems to split into one part that is primarily attending to the healing process and another part that simply remains in touch with events in the environment.

☐ 45. My mental perception seems clearer.

☐ 46. My thought processes seem to spring from intuitional insight rather than rationality.

☐ 47. I have no thoughts.

☐ 48. My thought processes seem to slow down.

☐ 49. I have thoughts, but I don't attend to them unless they relate to the healee and the Therapeutic Touch process.

☐ 50. My thoughts stop, and intuitions, images, and impressions take over.

☐ 51. I recognize imbalances in the healee's field.

☐ 52. I am aware of consciously directing my attention inward in order to center myself as I start the process.

☐ 53. My sense of concentration increases.

☐ 54. I am more aware of my inner being.

☐ 55. I am not aware of time.

☐ 56. I feel as if time stops.

☐ 57. I feel as if time slows down.

☐ 58. I feel as if time speeds up.

☐ 59. I feel that all personality patterns of the healee disappear, and all I see is his or her inner beauty.

☐ 60. I feel unified with the healee.

☐ 61. My body feels like an expanding mass of energy.

☐ 62. I feel as if my body is dissolving away and I am becoming boundless.

☐ 63. I experience my body as a continuous flow of energy rather than a set of distinct parts.

☐ 64. My cognitive processes seem to step into the background and become secondary to a more intuitive process of knowledge.

☐ 65. Parts of my body not actively involved in the Therapeutic Touch process feel heavy or nonexistent.

☐ 66. I have a feeling of being united with the external environment.

☐ 67. I have a sense of my own wholeness beyond my personality.

☐ 68. I am aware of a part of my being that is verbally or intuitively supplying me with knowledge of how best to direct energies to the healee's field.

CHAPTER 3

1. L.A. Govinda, *Foundations of Tibetan Mysticism* (London: Rider and Company, 1969), 116.

2. A. Avalon, *The Serpent Power* (Madras: Ganesh and Co., 1964).

3. C.W. Leadbeater, *The Chakras* (Wheaton, IL: Theosophical Publishing House, 1974).

4. D. Kunz, *The Personal Aura* (Wheaton, IL: Theosophical Publishing House, 1991).

5. D. Krieger, *Living the Therapeutic Touch: Healing as a Lifestyle* (New York: Dodd-Mead, 1987; distributed by Quest Books).

6. D. Krieger, *Therapeutic Touch: How to Use Your Hands to Help or to Heal* (New York: Prentice Hall Press, 1979).

7. Krieger, *Living the Therapeutic Touch*, 107-110, 157-187.

CHAPTER 4

1. D. Krieger, "Therapeutic Touch During Childbirth Preparation by the Lamaze Method and Its Relation to Marital Satisfaction and State Anxiety of the Married Couple" (Nursing Research Emphasis Grant for Doctoral Programs, U.S. Public Health Service, #NU-00833-02, Proceedings Research Day of Sigma Theta Tau, Upsilon Chapter, New York University, November 7, 1984).

2. D. Krieger, "Humanistic Models in a High-Tech World" (The Harry S. Truman Distinguished Lecturer award address, Avila College, Kansas City, MO, April 14, 1986).

3. H.R. Pagels, *The Cosmic Code: Quantum Physics as the Language of Nature* (New York: Simon and Schuster, 1982).

4. J. Woodruffe, *The Serpent Fire* (Madras: Ganesh, 1964), 105.

5. M. Eliade, *Yoga: Immortality and Freedom* (Princeton: Princeton University Press, 1969), 246.

6. W.Y. Evans-Wentz, *Tibet's Great Yogi Milarepa* (London: Oxford University Press, 1959), ix.

7. S. Karagulla and D. Kunz, *The Chakras and the Human Energy Field* (Wheaton, IL: Theosophical Publishing House, 1989).

8. L.A. Govinda, *Creative Meditation and Multidimensional Consciousness* (Wheaton, IL: Theosophical Publishing House, 1976), 71.

9. Karagulla and Kunz, *The Chakras and the Human Energy Field*.

10. D. Kunz, *The Personal Aura* (Wheaton, IL: Theosophical Publishing House, 1991).

11. L.K. Yu, *The Secret of Chinese Meditation* (London: Rider, 1964).

12. G. Krishna, *Kundalini: The Evolutionary Energy in Man* (Berkeley: Shambala, 1970).

13. Kunz, *The Personal Aura*.

14. D. Krieger, "The Relationship of Touch, with Intent to Help or Heal, to Subjects' In-vivo Hemoglobin Values: A Study in Personalized Interaction" (Proceedings, American Nurses Association 9th Nursing Research Conference, San Antonio, TX, March 21-23, 1973), 39-78.

15. D. Krieger, "Therapeutic Touch: The Imprimatur of Nursing," *American Journal of Nursing* 75 (1975): 784-787.

16. Krieger, "The Relationship of Touch."

CHAPTER 5

1. M. Dellas and E.L. Gauer, "Identification of Creativity: The Individual," *Psychol. Bull.* 73 (1970): 55-73.

2. Krieger, "Therapeutic Touch During Childbirth Preparation."

3. J.F. Chanes and T.X. Barber, "Acupuncture Analysis: A 6-Factor Theory," *Psychoenergetic Sys.* 1 (1974): 11-20.

4. E.H. Hale, "A study of the relationship between Therapeutic Touch and the anxiety of hospitalized patients" (unpublished doctoral dissertation, Texas Women's University, 1986).

5. P. Heidt, "An investigation of the effects of Therapeutic Touch on anxiety in hospitalized patients" (unpublished doctoral dissertation, New York University, 1979).

6. B.S. Parkes, "Therapeutic Touch as an intervention to reduce anxiety in elderly hospitalized patients" (unpublished doctoral dissertation, University of Texas, 1986).

7. J. Quinn, "An investigation of the effects of Therapeutic Touch done without physical contact on state anxiety of hospitalized patients" (unpublished doctoral dissertation, New York University, 1982).

8. E.D. Abravanel and E.A. King, *Dr. Abravanel's Body Type Program for Health and Fitness* (New York: Bantam Books, 1988).

9. M.R. Gach, *Acupressure's Potent Points: A Guide for Self Care for Common Ailments* (New York: Bantam Books, 1990).

10. R.S. Ryan, *The Fine Art of Recuperation: A Guide to Surviving and Thriving After Illness, Accident or Surgery* (Los Angeles: Jeremy Tarcher, Inc., 1989).

11. W.H. Hessam et al., *Consumer Reports Books: Guide to Income Tax Preparation (1991 edition)*, 256.

CHAPTER 6

1. J.R.M. Kunz and A.J. Finkel, eds., *The American Medical Association Family Medical Guide* (New York: Random House, 1987), 66-232.

2. Kunz, *The Personal Aura*.

3. R. Weber, *Dialogues with Scientists and Saints* (London: Routledge and Kegan Paul, 1986).

ABOUT THE AUTHOR

Dr. Krieger's life has been called a paradox: She has lived simultaneously in two worlds, and each world has bestowed upon her many honors. In the world of academia, she is professor emerita, New York University, and has been at the leading edge of research, theory development, and the clinical implementation of healing practices as a humane professional intervention.

In 1972, together with her colleague Dora Kunz, Dr. Krieger developed Therapeutic Touch, a contemporary interpretation of several ancient healing practices. They specifically developed Therapeutic Touch as an extension of professional skills for persons in the health field. Since 1984, when research by Dr. Krieger demonstrated both its feasibility and safety, Therapeutic Touch has been adapted for all people—children and adolescents as well as adults. Therapeutic Touch has now been taught in more than eighty colleges and universities in the United States and in sixty-seven foreign countries. In the world of alternative and collaborative healing modes, Therapeutic Touch is an acknowledged pioneer, for it has been consistently taught in fully accredited college and university curricula since 1975, an historical first.

Dr. Krieger's personal life reflects the far-flung scope of her interests. Her hobbies include French intensive organic gardening, mountain climbing, wood carving, rock collecting, reading ancient petroglyphs, and rebuilding old stone fences. She supports life-affirmative activities such as the humane protection of all endangered flora and fauna (including human beings at risk), and world-level coordinated, sustainable agricultural practices.